How Your Moral Self Affects Health and Humanity

Andre Antao

Copyright © 2025 Andre Antao

All rights reserved.

ISBN: 979-8-9870743-1-2

DEDICATION

In memory of my brother,

Sanford 1957-2018

CONTENTS

INTRODUCTION	1
TAKING THE MORAL-SELF PULSE OF OUR TIMES	6
THE MORAL ASPECT OF PERSONHOOD	26
POSTMODERN WORLD IMPACT ON MORAL SELF	53
WHAT COMPLICATES OUR MORAL SELF	87
HOW MORAL SELF DEVELOPS IN OUR PERSONHOOD	124
CONCLUSION	164

INTRODUCTION

Today, society often overlooks the moral core of personhood. There is a tendency to prioritize physical and social appearances over inner virtues. Showing strength through appearance rather than character has become common. Higher ideals, noble life purposes, integrity, and character are no longer widely regarded as essential personal qualities. Many people avoid confronting their deep personality traits and hide moral flaws, neglecting the importance of the moral self in shaping our humanity.

Every day, we try to maintain a public image focused on saving face rather than being authentic. Many adopt a false self as if it were their true self. However, without paying attention to our true self, we often only pretend to display virtues and hide our moral core, or, in the worst cases, become dishonest. When disconnected from our authentic self, we tend to be unclear or delusional about our identity. Today, we often fail to show the signs of psychological, emotional, and social maturity that define real personhood or lack a sense of a whole self.

In our daily interactions, people often seem unaware or confused about their true identity. When disconnected from the real self, their sense of identity becomes disorganized, unclear, and chaotic. This indicates that without a clear purpose for the moral self, the true self is overshadowed by the pseudo-self.

Anthropologically and psychologically, the moral self is the foundation of a person's identity. One's moral self is not only linked to individual health and well-being but also connected to the health and well-being of society and humanity. Health experts assert that the moral self influences the level of moral health in individuals and that moral health is crucial for improving overall health in all aspects. Contemporary social and cultural critics contend that society's health and welfare decline when people have low levels of moral health.

Evidence from life shows that the deviant and harmful moral self defines what it means to be human in postmodern times. In our society, people's behaviors are becoming increasingly cruel. This is evident every day in heinous crimes, vicious murders, corrupt practices, exploitation of the poor and powerless, violence against the vulnerable, and brutally inhumane treatment of others.

We live in a world increasingly shaped by evidence of a harmful and deviant moral self that destroys human life. Persistent social issues like illicit drug use, gun violence, mental health problems, and frequent brutal violence reflect a moral self that is becoming more stubborn and committed to pursuing harmful, inhumane, and evil actions. Everyday concerns such as mental and physical health issues, abusive relationships, the subjugation of the weak and powerless, and social inequalities are connected to moral and spiritual factors rather than just mental and social causes.

This is a challenging time in human history. We live amidst geopolitical, economic, cultural, and social instability. Around the world, it is characterized by warring nations, rebel groups, and terrorist organizations fighting for control; despots misusing their political power; and fanatical regimes committing genocide and ethnic cleansing. There are also horrific acts of terrorism happening at local, national, and international levels, along with an increasing number of localized and national anarchist movements.

This does not indicate moral health. Instead, many obvious signs of moral sickness are visible at local, national, and global levels, leading to concerning consequences for humanity.

In our world, only a few individuals develop a fully mature moral self. Most tend to remain trapped within a fixed, rigid moral identity. According to the latest research in neuromorality, a mature moral self can form through moral consciousness. In contrast, the fixed moral self is shaped by the standards, controls, and ideals of traditional morality.

In modern times, the inflexible and unchanging moral self of individuals no longer accurately reflects current moral understanding, feelings, and behaviors. Every day, people often ignore laws, deny objective truths, violate human rights, and justify evil actions, all while remaining loyal to traditional morality. The moral self that guides people's actions impairs moral rationality at individual, societal, and global levels, making it more difficult to form clear moral judgments in our evolving moral landscape. This primarily weakens humanity's moral health and contributes to a declining moral climate worldwide.

People's moral self today is often more hindered than helped by loyalty to traditional morality. To become better humans, we need to eliminate moral conflicts and dilemmas in daily life, which stem from a static, rigid moral self. The declining moral environment worldwide reflects a static moral self that fails to help people change, grow, and evolve. Without developing a mature moral self driven by moral awareness, we lack the psychosocial maturity needed to form meaningful relationships in society that can improve the world.

An individual's capacity to cultivate, maintain, and uphold humaneness in today's world depends on the objectivity and rationality of a mature moral self. The mature self exhibits more than just concern for prosocial qualities and behaviors expected for human decency in society. It acts as the pathway to psychosocial maturity by championing the core principles of the common good, interdependence, and human solidarity, which are vital in our world.

Few people commit to developing the moral capacities of the moral self necessary in the postmodern world to handle moral dilemmas, challenges, and responsibilities. Clearly, the only way to be human today, as in the past, is by cultivating a mature moral self of personhood. This primarily occurs when we are willing to stay engaged in the lifelong process of self-evolution, which develops moral consciousness essential for maturing the moral self.

Today, both as individuals and as a society, we experience intense moral pain and suffering. The world around us shows more signs of moral sickness than moral health. The widespread moral sickness in our world exposes more about people's corrupt moral selves than any other aspect of human life.

Moral pain and suffering are primary sources of new social issues, problems, and evils unique to the postmodern era. The decline in moral well-being in modern society underscores the importance of focusing on one's moral self. The typical moral self of people today is less effective than it needs to be for growth, improvement, and maintaining moral health, which has wide-ranging implications for human life.

This book offers a scholarly analysis of the moral self, which is prominent in the postmodern world, and its impact on personal and collective health and humanity. It aims to educate readers about the importance of caring for one's moral self and promoting moral health, both to improve individual and societal well-being and to support the health and welfare of society and humanity.

The book starts by evaluating the state of the moral self, emphasizing its condition in our society. Its aim is to help readers identify the moral self as a vital human experience that greatly influences life. The book then examines the conceptual foundation of the moral self in personhood, which many overlook, to promote a clear understanding of its existential role and its intricate impact on all facets of human life. Analyzing the moral self improves the understanding of moral sickness in modern times as a matter of existential health.

Most of the book examines how the postmodern world impacts the moral self for both current and future generations. By exploring the unique effects of postmodernity on modern human culture, values, sense of self, and health issues, the book highlights problems caused by dependence on institutional moral rationality, which dominates today's society. It shows how this influence shapes people's daily thoughts and behaviors. Then, by analyzing individuals' everyday work self-concept and self-identity within modern society, the book considers the moral self that guides daily life for ordinary people. It stresses how these daily self-concepts and self-identities are vital to the well-being of individuals, society, the planet, and humanity.

The main goal of the book is to highlight the moral self that develops through moral consciousness, rather than when it is shaped by conventional morality. Almost everyone claims to embody the moral self, which is influenced by moral systems instead of moral awareness. The reader will gain a clearer understanding of how the postmodern world makes it difficult to grow in moral consciousness as a better, more effective, more relevant, and more purposeful way to address conflicts, dilemmas, challenges, and problems in today's moral landscape.

At a minimum, the book should provide the reader with insight into a topic that is critically important for personal healthcare but is rarely discussed. It will help the reader explore how this fundamental human phenomenon – the moral self of personhood – influences not only individual health but also creates ripple effects on the broader world we live in, reflected through everyday experiences, both ordinary and extraordinary, in our times.

TAKING THE MORAL-SELF PULSE OF OUR TIMES

If we evaluated the moral character of our era, only a few would demonstrate the human decency, integrity, and character that everyone once aspired to. Few people start to embody the higher ideals, values, attitudes, and habits that reflect a richer, nobler, and more shining life. The lack of such role models is a unique and troubling aspect of the postmodern world.

In modern society, life experiences often show that people generally lack the self-control of the wise, virtuous, and high-minded. We interact with individuals who are habitually impulsive, imprudent, and rude. An average person mishandles the natural flow of harmful and dangerous thoughts, feelings, and actions. The unfiltered thoughts and impulses cause people to become overly reactive and often lose control of themselves.

In modern society, we observe people leaning toward vileness, viciousness, and what is repulsive, rather than the calmness of the civilized and prudence of the wise. Usually, daily behaviors reveal that people's minds are shaped by crude ideas that block or hinder moral goals in life. The everyday moral reasoning often serves to justify oneself and deny moral responsibility.

In modern society, experiences like duplicity, scandals, corruption, scams, crimes, violence, human trafficking, and evil often define what it means to be human. There seems to be no way to eliminate the forces of evil in our world. The evidence is clear in how easily we give in to what is unethical, immoral, illegal, and even inhumane. The devilish erodes what is human in each of us.

Accustomed to the dehumanizing aspects within us, we struggle to understand what it truly means to be human in others. Desensitized to our inhumane tendencies, we have lost control over heinous crimes and brutal killings. As we become used to a world filled with violence, we kill fellow humans no differently than hunters pursue trophies. The violent deaths in modern society reveal that the remnants of the "animal" inside us are overtaking our humanity.

In modern society, people struggle to empathize and understand what truly makes us human, both in ourselves and in others. We go through life with less of our human side exposed than we might realize. Experts in human behavior say that the brain mechanisms responsible for being other-focused are gradually becoming disrupted.[1] Now, it seems to be only wishful thinking for fellow humans to find what is human in themselves and others.

In modern society, pets tend to respond more to our human needs for comfort, honesty, and well-being. What stands out today is that qualities once seen as human traits—such as kindness, politeness, honesty, tolerance, and loyalty—are now increasingly valued in the culture of keeping animals as pets. This may explain why many people consider pets part of the family.

In modern society, people often feel a deep unease with who they are and who they pretend to be. It's similar to what children on the verge of adulthood experience. They not only feel uncertain about their true selves but also confuse others about who they really are. They find themselves trapped in a false sense of identity, living in a make-believe world of fantasies—people who feel unsettled inside lack a strong moral foundation.

---

[1] Filkowski, M., Cochran, R., Hass, B. Altruistic behavior: mapping responses in the brain Neurosci Neuroecon. Nov. 2016

In modern society, people often rest on a fragile foundation of fantasies, insecurities, and vulnerabilities, which leads to self-destruction and a loss of coherence. Modernity has shaped individuals with adaptable personalities, characterized by cold indifference and aloofness. It most clearly reveals a weak moral sense of personhood. The darkened mind and an impassive spirit generally define people's moral character today. In everyday life, people have no hesitation in engaging in cruelty, corruption, perverse behavior, reprobate deeds, and other evil acts. The depravity of humanity in postmodern times exposes more of the darkness and evil within individuals.

In modern society, many people see unethical and immoral behavior as a survival tactic. No one seems concerned about wrongdoing or evil acts, regardless of their severity to themselves and others. The current generation has a carefree attitude and is even unafraid of being held accountable for heinous or illegal acts. People often and habitually turn toward the egregious, deplorable, devilish, and outrageous. We find ourselves unable to focus on higher purposes, virtuous living, or the common good.

Human life in the postmodern world faces moral chaos, disorder, and conflicts. Humanity is gradually losing moral integrity. The poor moral environment reflects a decline in overall moral health. Literature experts note that today's human landscape indicates an underdeveloped and ineffective "moral brain." Scientists emphasize a brain region vital for moral emotions, motivation, and decision-making, known as the "moral brain." The frequent occurrence of severe problematic behaviors suggests a disruption in the functioning of the human brain, including its higher cognitive and emotional functions.

In the postmodern world, people realize that eliminating the moral framework of self-centeredness is impossible. We often operate from an unpredictable, erratic mindset characterized by self-absorption, egotism, and hedonism. Most individuals struggle with self-discipline and self-control. The moral self that people promote allows for self-deception and hinders self-denial. Without a mature moral self, we cannot become the best version of ourselves or develop human qualities that enhance relationship patterns for social cohesion and a humane world.

We can better understand the moral self's pulse in our era by examining the factors that influence its development in the postmodern world. We will analyze the evolution of the moral self from the perspectives of (1) the ineffectiveness of traditional morality and legal systems, (2) the denial of objective truth, (3) the tendency toward self-deception, (4) the dominance of modern technology, and (5) the toxicity of "quick-fix" solutions.

Ineffectiveness of Traditional Moral and Legal Systems

On a global scale, it's clear that we are living in a world morally in decline. Humanity seems to be in the late stages of moral corruption. This is often shown through dishonest politicians and their divisiveness, hypocritical religious leaders with double standards, greedy corporate executives, increasing military spending by competing nations, genocide by oppressive regimes, the effects of global terrorism, and man-made natural disasters, along with serious threats to the planet's future.

Additionally, every day, we hear about or face evil on a smaller scale: violence, crime, suicide, homicide, dysfunctional families, drug abuse, and more. We often encounter the charlatan, the trickster, the scoundrel, and the humbug, and have come to expect and even respect them. These are not signs of moral health!

Furthermore, we live in a world where people are treated no differently than objects for personal gain and victory. Utilitarian behaviors are normalized in our interactions to the point that fellow humans are seen as disposable things. Today, we seldom meet people who are less self-centered and more caring about others.

Sadly, today's moral climate increasingly leads us to question whether a principled, virtuous, and noble life is even possible. It reveals that society's legal, moral, and ethical systems don't motivate people to achieve higher levels of personhood. We adopt a moral self mainly to avoid judgment and condemnation, seek social acceptance, and publicly display human decency to maintain a good standing with society.

Conventional morality and legal systems, which often involve following widely accepted social norms and expectations, are proving to be insufficient in promoting holistic health and the well-being of the entire person. People feel pressured to conform to these norms even if they conflict with their personal values and desires, which can lead to anxiety, stress, and a lowered sense of self-worth. Societal expectations may dictate how individuals are "supposed" to feel in certain situations, resulting in emotional dissonance when genuine feelings do not match these expectations. Experts warn that hiding true emotions to fit social norms can cause chronic stress and emotional burnout.[2]

Evidence from the postmodern era shows that traditional morality and legal systems alone are not enough to navigate a rapidly changing world. While scientific and technological advances bring many benefits, they also create new problems. Our society faces complex moral issues, particularly when individuals act morally to meet external standards without aligning their instincts and reasoning with their overall health, lifestyle, or society's well-being. This disconnect weakens the higher self's sense of personhood, as modern morality and law often clash with innate moral instincts, hindering genuine moral growth.

The most common stereotype of the moral self involves rules of morality and legality. This view suggests that people can develop a strong tendency to "be moral" without necessarily "acting moral." Often, we do not respond with the appropriate moral actions in urgent moral situations but act

---

[2] Bhandari, S. Mental Health Effects of Unrealistic Expectations. WebMed; Feb. 2025

only in ways dictated by external moral principles and ideals. We are unable to develop a broad perspective in the moral realm to consider alternative moral rationalities. Our way of being "moral" in everyday conflicts and dilemmas reveals a lack of clear moral purpose, an inability to uphold higher ideals, insensitivity, moral numbness, poor tolerance and compassion, and a deficiency in altruism and magnanimity. In short, we are depriving ourselves of the human consciousness that allows us to reach the heights of sublime human nature, as seen in higher-order personhood and holistic selfhood.

With little or no awareness of our moral self, we go through daily life more mechanically than genuinely. Without understanding our moral being, we become disconnected from the actual experience of existence. We deny the self-truth that is vital for self-transparency and authenticity. Every day, we support, participate in, and even contribute to a culture of deception, fantasies, and illusions. Consequently, we live with many illusions about who we are and the purpose of our human existence.

We might think we belong to a generation that is remarkably knowledgeable because of scientific and technological progress. However, realistically, science and technology have just fictionalized the natural order of human life. We tend to see the fictional products of human creation as human achievements. Relying solely on science and technology in the postmodern world leads us to overlook the deeper human vitality essential for growth in our profound humanity.

Achievements in science and technology haven't helped people outgrow narrow-mindedness, biased self-views, and limited worldviews. While groundbreaking scientific achievements demonstrate the impressive creative power of the human brain, they also risk stripping away what it means to be human in a postmodern world. Although modern science is rapidly advancing in its understanding of the human mind and behavior, we still grapple with irrationality, impulsiveness, and inhumanity. Superstition and magical thinking still influence the human psyche.

Claims of progress in human life haven't helped us build the moral self capable of perspectives, attitudes, and values that override short-term impulses and desires. Every day, people are hurt by their out-of-control self-deception and are flooded with self-delusional ideas. We chase illusory life goals and tend to feel invincible until tragedy hits – as it inevitably does, no matter how unexpected.

Propensity to Deny Objective Truth

Anything that harms moral integrity in everyday life suggests that people are eroding the truth. This is happening so widely that it seems people believe there is no choice but to deny the truth. It has become common for people to distort, withhold, spin, tell half-truths, invent falsehoods, obscure the truth with revisionist thinking and euphemisms, and propagate outright lies.

Perhaps, in today's world, denial, manipulation, and sabotage of the truth are clear signs of people's weak moral character. Everyday life experiences suggest that many individuals cannot imagine a better way to interact than through deception, manipulation, fraud, and scheming in their daily dealings. They don't believe others deserve fair, honest, and trustworthy treatment. The tendency to deny objective truth also makes us unwilling to recognize our self-truths, which, if acknowledged, could be therapeutic and deepen our sense of self, way of life, and our place in the world.

In our world, people have only a fragile connection to the truth. There is a denial of the very existence of objective truths. We have become accustomed to a culture of lying, cheating, evasiveness, and doing whatever it takes to avoid the truth. We accept falsehoods in personal relationships, social interactions, and living situations. Sometimes, it even happens that we lie to ourselves without realizing it. Worse yet, we can convince ourselves that our lies are the truth.

In a world that is undeniably diverse, internet culture has united people.

Today, the internet seems to be the only shared aspect of human life. However, everyday experiences show that the truth is often the first casualty of internet culture. Misinformation, disinformation, and twisted ideologies spread like a dangerous disease. People become entangled in the malicious intentions of strangers' deceitful lies. Moreover, the internet exposes everyone to manipulative algorithms that warp the truth. Ironically, while internet technology has significantly improved our quality of life, it has also distanced us from human virtues such as honesty, truth, integrity, character, respect, honor, and higher-order thinking.

The global culture not only dismisses but also obstructs and hinders people from seeking and sharing the objective truth. Denying the truth is so common in society that it is now even evident in the press. The news media, which everyone once trusted unwaveringly to honor truth, are now only known for delivering "news" rather than the truth. False news reports in the media and illegal postings on social media platforms overshadow human decency with the shadow of a darkened heart and a sick human spirit.

What are the implications of denying objective truth on people's moral selves, and what does it reveal about the state of moral identity in the postmodern world?

Denying objective truth, especially in moral issues, can significantly impact the moral self in various ways. It implies that many people think there are no universal, lasting, and unchanging moral truths and purposes in human life. This suggests that the moral self is rooted in personal or cultural preferences, which can hinder our efforts to develop higher-level personhood and foster human solidarity for the common good.

In the postmodern world, the denial of objective truths has led to moral viewpoints being regarded as equally valid, regardless of their adverse effects on human well-being. Moral relativism establishes moral standards without considering the harm inflicted on others. It has made resolving moral conflicts and dilemmas more difficult on a personal level. Moreover, moral relativism fosters moral disagreements within society. Globally, people's differing moral goals have contributed to social fragmentation and disintegration. Without access to objective truth, individuals' moral identities tend to prioritize self-interest over the common good, myopic worldviews over comprehensive ones, and exclusiveness over inclusiveness in social relationships.

People's purely subjective truths make them less accountable for their actions because they trust their own decisions. In everyday life, this results in a lack of moral responsibility for our duties toward the well-being of others, society, or humanity. The moral reasoning that guides the moral self often leads to behaviors that harm others and disrupt social order. Without a clear moral framework based on objective truth, it becomes difficult to handle complex moral dilemmas. People live with unresolved moral conflicts and urgent ethical issues. The moral confusion among individuals makes it hard for them to set clear goals or standards for moral growth and reform in society.

The tendency to deny objective truth in the moral realm weakens the strong moral foundation that helps people identify and call out wrongdoing and evil for what they are. It encourages subjective values that prevent individuals from perceiving and admitting morally wrong actions and behaviors. When transparent and objective moral standards are absent, it results in a state of "post-truth," where judgments are based on personal opinions rather than facts. In our world, this occurs constantly, and we have become desensitized to it. This is especially clear in wars fought without any objective justification. Meanwhile, innocent victims suffer terrible consequences caused by reprehensible morals.

The erosion of trust and social bonds can occur when people engage in deception, even if transparent lies are uncovered. Those who lie may assume others are dishonest, fostering distrust even toward honest individuals in their social circles. Experts state that people who view themselves as less trustworthy are less likely to form strong social connections and might see others as untrustworthy, creating a cycle of mistrust.[3]

Dishonesty, regardless of intent, can damage a person's moral integrity and impede the development of moral health and social well-being.

In summary, rejecting objective truth, especially in moral matters, can harm an individual's moral self, their ability to reason morally, and their motivation to act rightly. It erodes the objective basis for condemning harmful actions and leads to negative effects on social relationships. It also diminishes people's capacity to trust each other and hampers human solidarity.

Propensity for Self-Deception

Unable to envision objective truth, we have cultivated a culture of self-denial and self-delusions, chasing after illusions. We struggle to grasp the existential truth of who we are and the reality of what we do because of who we are. People lack moral clarity and a clear vision for a better version of themselves and are indifferent or unaware of the goodness beneath their self-perceptions. We also lack the courage to recognize whatever may be evil in us for what it is. On a global scale, people seem shattered and distraught, forced to hide their "self-truths" and confront the inner reality of the "real self."

In our society, "being evil" and "doing evil" are increasingly regarded as usual in the pursuit of the "good life." This trend is so widespread that it gradually causes lasting damage to individuals' moral selves. Evidence of this appears daily in societies worldwide through alarming rates of mental health issues, drug addiction, violence, crimes, suicides, and homicides, as well as the rise of communal tensions, social unrest, terrorism, and geopolitical conflicts that lower the quality of life for ordinary people.

Experts highlight that everyday self-deception clouds people's ability to evaluate situations, especially concerning moral issues and judgments,

---

[3] Sprigings, S., Brown, C., Brinke, L. Deception is associated with reduced social connection. Communication Psychology (Vol. 1); 2023

accurately.[4] Self-deception often results in justifying harmful actions, enabling us to convince ourselves that these actions are morally right. It allows individuals to mitigate the effects and consequences of wrongdoing and evil. Self-deception reflects the moral self in our society, showing that people not only distort the impact of their actions but also how they judge others, leading to biased assessments and unfair treatment.

Self-deception can prevent us from recognizing our mistakes and learning from them. By ignoring the truth about their flaws and shortcomings, people might miss opportunities for personal growth and moral development. This can result in stagnation in moral progress and a cycle of repeated harmful behaviors and declining moral health. Research indicates that while self-deception might offer temporary relief from negative feelings, it can ultimately cause anxiety, guilt, and internal conflict. Researchers argue that the effort required to maintain a self-deceptive facade can be psychologically exhausting and unsustainable.[5]

Although self-deception is a standard part of human life in society, there's always a lingering feeling that something about who we are, what we do, and where we're headed in life seems off. Still, we resist facing the actual reality of our human condition. Instead, we create ideas about human nature and the purpose of life to avoid confronting harsh self-truths. We hold onto false beliefs about our identity and the meaning of life, building an illusory world filled with childish fantasies about ourselves and the world. Today, it feels as if the human being is just a bag of skin full of illusions.

People often lack a deep understanding of what it truly means to be human. Few realize that being human is fundamentally linked to moral nature. Even fewer see that one's moral health is closely connected to one's humanity.

---

[4] The Encyclopedia of Applied Ethics, Second Edition; 2012.
[5] Preuter, S., Jaeger, B., Stel, M. The cost of lying: Consequences of telling lies on liar's self-esteem and affect. British Journal of Social Psychology; 2023.

The common tendency to deceive ourselves creates a mindset that downplays the importance of higher personhood and holistic selfhood; we must genuinely be human in a postmodern society. Many of us deny that the poorer quality of human life today is influenced by declining moral health in people. It is also rare to consider that moral health affects other aspects of health, including spiritual, mental, social, and physical realms. Most importantly, the collective decline in moral health presents the greatest threat to human existence now.

In today's society, higher-order personhood often gives in to what harms human nature and diminishes human dignity. Human qualities, virtues, and decency fade under the influence of irrational impulses and illogical self-beliefs. Every day, people's intolerance, anger, hatred, aggression, vengeance, violence, and evil acts are often more expressions of self-hatred. People struggle to find the "inner space" needed to uncover their self-truths, overcome self-deceptions, and achieve self-acceptance and self-love, ultimately hindering their ability to become a better version of themselves. It can be said that the human tragedy of our time is the loss of genuine self-love and self-care.

We often avoid truly understanding ourselves. At the same time, we struggle to be free from moral pain and suffering. While existential suffering is unavoidable, moral pain is not. In daily life, it's clear there is a basic human craving for rich experiences of all kinds. This demonstrates that, despite our technological advances, we still desire a more meaningful human life. On some level of self-awareness, people want a better moral self to fulfill the longing to be better human beings.

In conclusion, while self-deception might seem like a way to cope with challenging situations, it ultimately harms the moral self and well-being by distorting reality, eroding trust, blocking personal growth, and preventing people from living authentically. The lack of authenticity in individuals leads many to feel emptiness and dissatisfaction with themselves and life.

Dominance of Modern Technology

Furthermore, in the high-tech world, we often misunderstand what is true about the human person. Today, human reality is tangled in complex technological layers. People have a poor grasp of themselves because they cannot see the true potential of human nature. The neglect of what it takes to be human has led to the creation of many personas. We hide from the truth about our real, unique inner selves. People often mask or distance themselves from their true selves, the genuine individuals they are inside.

Technology is a tool that can be used for good or bad, and its impact on moral well-being depends on how it is designed, used, and governed. Technology has a complex and multifaceted influence on the moral self in modern society, which requires ongoing research and careful consideration of its implications for moral health. Existing research shows that modern technological advances have had both positive and negative effects on people's moral selves.[6]

Overall, modern technologies enhance connectivity and communication, increase awareness of social, political, and global issues, and can promote empathy in decision-making and behavior. However, digital addiction may lead to mental health problems such as depression, loneliness, and even suicidal thoughts, particularly among young adults. The rapid pace and broad reach of technology can also spread misinformation, fueling polarization and distrust. The same tools that support positive moral choices can also be used for harmful actions like hate speech and misinformation on social media. Moreover, unequal access to technology can exacerbate existing inequalities in areas such as education, employment, and social inclusion.

In a world that celebrates human productivity, people avoid confronting their true selves by staying constantly busy; they replace being with

---

[6] <u>Information Technology and Moral Values</u>. Stanford Encyclopedia of Philosophy, 2018.

doing. We have sacrificed human virtues like decency, personal integrity, and noble character for self-delusional ideas and self-serving schemes. Even worse, many individuals have become like "human robots."

This is reflected in our modern digital culture. Almost everyone spends nearly every waking moment using tech gadgets and devices. This applies to both literate and illiterate, young and old. As humans, we have become roughly robotic, acting as little more than extensions of our technology, which leads us toward self-alienation and social isolation, fueled by a false belief in an "undefeatable power" within us.

The "human robot" represents the new reality of our times, exercising power with cold logic and indifference. We can better understand this new human phenomenon, created through the illusion of "undefeatable power," by examining the concept of the machine. It comes from the word mechos. The etymology of "machine" shows its close connection to deception, as the lever in a machine is designed to cheat gravity when lifting heavy objects.

The Greek word mechos means a trap set by a clever person. It comes from the ancient magh, which is reflected in the German words Macht and mogen, both of which mean might. From this German root, the English word might function both as a noun for power and as a verb indicating a faint possibility or unreality. Based on this origin, we can conclude that the "human-robot" only gains self-identity through the apparent power we possess.

The imaginary power of human-robot interactions diminishes the metaphysical aspects of humans and distorts the individual's sense of self. The moral and spiritual aspects are essential human realities and form the foundation of human nature. No machine can replicate these realities or embody what it means to be human. The selfhood of human robots challenges what it means to be human by shifting core human realities within a person.

Modern technologies have significant impacts on the moral health of individuals, societies, and the world. The moral shifts caused by technology are drastically changing how we think, feel, and act in the postmodern age. The social systems created by technology often end up being harmful and corrupting. There is a weak distinction between what is "morally valuable"—worth pursuing, promoting, and cherishing—and what is not, which should be ignored, undermined, or minimized. The moral reasoning of today is often based not on objective ideas of good or bad, right or wrong, but on self-interest and personal priorities. As a result, what supports the moral purpose of the common good and human solidarity is often distorted or undermined.

A deeper look into the unseen effects of scientific and technological progress reveals today how we navigate life, connecting more like human robots than truly human beings. These human robots are so heavily influenced by technology that their perceptions prevent them from recognizing their own soulless, emotionless, and often manipulative behaviors. We interact as human robots who tempt, deceive, and take advantage of others to serve our interests. Every day, we realize—sometimes painfully—that people tend to be only who they believe they are or want others to think they are.

The technological world has made us more machine-like, pushing us every day toward a false sense of self. We often prioritize superficiality over good causes, common sense, and deeper insights, and we fail to approach issues with calm, rational, and realistic thinking. Lacking epistemic stances on moral reasoning and motivations, it becomes harder for us to exercise sound judgment, impartiality, and accountability. We care less about others deserving fair, just, and trustworthy treatment. As a result, in today's world, desperate cries for truth, justice, and human respect often go unheard. We show cold indifference and aloofness in human interactions.

The signs of the times suggest we may be heading toward the frightening outcomes of our actions. By neglecting the moral and spiritual core of human nature, it's clear that humanity has become fragmented and muted. Despite all the progress, achievements, and comforts in our world, people everywhere still feel unfulfilled. They seek inner freedom and peace that "self-contentment" alone offers. It shows us that, as a whole, humanity lives without tapping into the potential of moral human nature. Wise and prudent voices make clear calls condemning the unchecked human creations of our era as, at best, illusions and, at worst, catastrophic. They warn that the vanity of collective behaviors is a destructive approach for the human race.

Public opinion about humanity's moral health indicates that we are living in very troubling times and a dangerous world. These ideas also reflect in nearly everyone's fears and anxieties. The daily existential angst people face shows an unsettling state of humanity in the postmodern world. The turmoil in the world mainly highlights the declining moral climate on a global scale and the intense moral suffering of humanity.

Toxicity of "Quick Fixes" Solutions

Many attribute humanity's low level of moral health today to the influence of the culture of "quick-fix" solutions. The global culture of individualism, materialism, consumerism, and hedonism promotes a tendency toward "quick-fix" solutions, which significantly impact the moral self in modern society. The rhythm of the moral self is influenced by triggers and stimuli from the worldwide sociocultural environment, which shape people's moral perceptions and can lead to misunderstandings, illusions, and lax permissiveness.

Global cultural phenomena primarily shape people's life priorities and goals. In today's global culture, many see no alternative to a self-centered lifestyle. The pursuit of pleasure fuels daily self-focused behaviors. Hedonism drives individuals with an acquisitive mindset to chase more wealth, fame, and power, often regardless of the cost. They are driven by aspirations to become rich and famous for their own sake. Almost everyone indulges in the fantasy of being the luckiest, happiest, and greatest. Few express a desire to pursue higher ideals or leave a virtuous legacy. Human solidarity and the common good are rarely intentionally embraced in the pursuits of ordinary people.

The relentless pursuit of self-centered goals in life has become like blinders that people find difficult, if not impossible, to remove. The cultural mindset of egotism and insatiable greed not only encourages wrong-minded behaviors but also fosters sociopathic and psychopathic tendencies in individuals. Experts say that increased individualism and a decrease in empathy contribute to antisocial behaviors in modern society.[7] Health professionals believe that sociopathic and psychopathic personality traits exist on a spectrum and are increasingly common among the general population.

Despite humanity's prosperity, impressive achievements, modern comforts, luxuries, and scientific rationalism, people still see their lives as fragile and challenging. Many in today's society experience deep despair and a sense of meaninglessness. Cultural critics see the destructive influence of hedonism's dominance in postmodern culture as shaping a harmful moral self. We exhibit behaviors driven by moral irrationality, which weaken higher ideals and life's greater purposes. The pursuit of the "good life" in modern society is primarily based on an immoral or amoral mindset. The moral stance and capacity for happiness that people seek aren't helping them achieve the "freedoms" they also desire in life.

In the postmodern world, people regularly breathe in and exhale toxic values and attitudes leaking from the cultural environment. Modernity trains us for quick-fix solutions, short-term rewards, and mind-numbing intoxications. For nearly everyone, self-fulfillment doesn't include a higher sense of what is good, right, just, and fair. We are used to living without a trace of human dignity and decency.

The relentless craving for "quick-fix" solutions in modern society has harmful effects on everyday moral behavior. "Quick-fixes" emphasize

---

[7] Waytz, A. & Gray, K. *Does Online Technology Make Us More or Less Sociable? A Preliminary Review and Call for Research.* Sage Journals (Vol. 13); 2018

immediate pleasure or relief without considering the long-term consequences. Experts warn that seeking instant gratification often causes people to make impulsive choices and poor decisions.[8] People who depend on quick-fix solutions weaken their ability to recognize and address real problems.

Research shows that when people make harmful decisions quickly, they tend to be more selfish. It highlights the moral state of our times, emphasizing personal beliefs, ideas, and whims over objective truth and value-based standards. It points to a clear self-centeredness in pursuing one's desires. The tendency for "quick-fix" solutions reveals an inadequate or even damaging moral self in a person. In daily life, it's clear that those who look for "quick-fix" solutions often ignore ethical guidelines and professional standards, risking harm or exploitation. Health professionals suggest that over time, this can lead to feelings of helplessness, lower self-confidence, and ultimately weaken self-regulation and personal growth.

Neuroscience shows that repeatedly choosing "quick-fixes" can create neural pathways that reinforce the behavior, making change more difficult. When we consistently engage in a behavior, like seeking a "quick-fix," our brain develops stronger neural networks related to that action. Relying on "quick-fixes" can lead to poor impulse control and decreased emotional regulation. Focusing on quick-fix benefits may cause us to overlook long-term social or environmental impacts. The core of this moral self suggests that overconfidence in our moral judgments often results in taking unnecessary risks that put others at risk.

In summary, relying on a "quick-fix" mentality often fosters moral issues by impairing the ability to see objective truth, weakening moral reasoning needed for addressing ethical dilemmas, and raising vulnerability to harmful

---

[8] Mehta, K. Why You Succumb to Instant Gratification – And the Easiest Way to Make Life Optimizing Choices. Forbes; Oct. 2022
Perlmutter, A. The Real Issue with Instant Gratification. Psychology Today; Sept. 2019

habits and addictions. This approach promotes immoral and unethical actions through immediate, selfish choices, frequently neglecting long-term outcomes.

So, what can be said about the pulse of our moral self during these times?

The pulse of the moral self in our times shows that the human tragedy in our postmodern world is that people are morally lost, confused, disoriented, and conflicted. We have plenty of everything in every possible way compared to past generations, yet we lack our true selves.

The pulse of the moral self in our times reveals people's underdeveloped moral sense, resulting in a poor ability to form relationships that help heal and improve individuals. People everywhere struggle to build secure, stable, and enriching relationships. Most have become used to and comfortable with relating in ways that seem fake and insincere, lacking depth and authenticity. Yet, at the same time, people long to be understood, cared for, and loved.

The pulse of the moral self today shows that in our short human life, we often waste time without real purpose. We vaguely recognize the fleeting nature of human existence. We think that staying busy is what will give us self-worth, security, and happiness. In chasing illusions of the "good life," we ignore the sensible, balanced, and holistic way of living.

The moral compass of our times suggests that the idea of the "good life" in the postmodern world weakens fundamental self-awareness and self-control. Rational thinking and wisdom often overshadow unpredictable and uncontrollable impulses. We tend to avoid confronting the full depth of our human suffering, which is intensified by moral pain. As a result, we are losing control over behaviors that threaten our hopes and aspirations for what it means to be human in the world.

The focus of the moral self today indicates that most of us lack true insight into who we are and why we're here. We tend to overlook the limited nature of human life and ignore the higher purpose in our lives; as a result, we miss out on the journey of self-evolution, moral growth, and the development of higher consciousness and holistic selfhood.

The pulse of the moral self in our times shows that people do not realize they are destined for immortality; they lack the vision of their immortality as the most significant human achievement. Only a few rarely show a desire to be immortal by living virtuous, honorable, and shining lives.

Finally, the moral pulse in our times reflects humanity's decline into aimlessness that urgently calls for the refinement of mental, moral, and spiritual habits. Together, we must be rooted in a strong inner foundation, with a more transparent and more solid understanding of values, goals, and motivations in daily life. We also need to overcome the delusions and illusions that have shaped our current human landscape.

THE MORAL ASPECT OF PERSONHOOD

The personhood of an individual is expressed across various dimensions. Each day, references are made to people's "physical self," "emotional self," "psychological self," "spiritual self," and "moral self." We understand that there are different aspects to a person's selfhood. The selfhood we acknowledge often shows that one or more components of personhood are coming forward. Usually, we do not give equal importance to all elements of personhood when shaping selfhood.

Natural law views personhood as a core human trait and a natural right. Humans are considered "natural persons" from birth to death because of their intellectual, aesthetic, moral, and spiritual capacities. What makes personhood uniquely human is that humans not only have innate mental, spiritual, and moral abilities but can also develop them. Although personhood has been controversially assigned to pets, animals, and robots, there is a growing agreement among experts in anthropology and zoology that it is a concept reserved exclusively for humans.

Personhood is not based on physical traits and cannot be reduced to the physical. It includes the whole person, covering both physical and non-physical aspects—mind, body, spirit, and social environment. The development of one's personhood is a continuous life process that involves bio-psycho-emotional growth. At the same time, it also entails the spiritual, moral, and social maturity of the individual. The overall result is the experience of the human personality.

Personhood refers to what is irreplaceable and reflects a person's individuality. It focuses on the uniqueness of an individual that makes them irreplaceable. From a psycho-anthropological perspective, personhood is the core, indivisible personal element closely connected to society and culture. The sense of personhood exists within internal psycho-emotional and mental processes, which are fundamentally relational.

The sense of personhood can only develop through relationships. To be a human person is to relate. The meaning of personhood always centers on relationships. We build our sense of personhood through our connections with ourselves, others, and the world. It arises from the perceptions we and others hold of us. The relational view of personhood shows that it results from a dialectical interplay of intentionality, meanings, values, and life experiences.

It is through relationships that we understand each other's personhood. These perceptions shape the self-concept, self-identity, and social image of a person. However, personhood always involves both autonomy and interdependence. Therefore, self-concept, self-identity, and social image are based on the freedom to choose, decide, and accept responsibility.

Humans are both individuals and social beings, inherently connected through their nature. The essence of human nature is defined by freedom and responsibility. These qualities are vital to a person's sense of identity. The development of personhood relies on an individual's freedom and responsibility as both a personal and social being. Human health and maturity are rooted in the personal freedom to make choices and the responsibility we bear toward ourselves and others.

The relational idea of personhood also explains human growth and health through relationships. It places health and well-being within a framework of relational responsibilities. The role of personhood in health is based on a relational foundation. This shows that human health is mainly a relational phenomenon.

Personhood is the most critical factor in all health efforts. As a multidisciplinary concept, personhood guides actions across physical, mental, social, moral, and spiritual domains. A person's sense of personhood determines the type of health work required. Modern health sciences state that a person's sense of identity directly influences the development, improvement, and maintenance of overall health.

Modern health sciences focus on personhood as a key principle of human health. Experts believe that developing personhood is linked to preserving life and health, caring with beneficence, maintaining relational integrity, respecting human rights and dignity, acting with truth and justice in society, and promoting human solidarity and global peace. All of these depend on the moral dimension of personhood.

Although often overlooked, the core human aspects of personhood—the moral and spiritual—serve as guiding principles for health. These vital spiritual and moral elements form the foundation of higher-level personhood. They promote behaviors that improve life and foster a sense of wholeness. Wholesome personhood arises from the strength of one's spiritual and moral capacities. Engaging with these core human aspects of personhood is essential for building and maintaining good health.

The inherent potential for spiritual and moral capacities is essential for nurturing one's sense of self. Without access to these potentials, it can lead to a gradual breakdown of personhood and self-identity. Developing these capacities enables a person to be truly whole. A holistic individual grows by cultivating innate spiritual and moral abilities. The holistic human engages in life with these spiritual and moral capacities.

The spiritual and moral aspects of personhood are vital for both individual and societal well-being. They are fundamental to human growth, healthcare efforts, and social progress. Society's and humanity's welfare depend more on these moral and spiritual qualities than on any other factor. Without highlighting the human spiritual and moral core, progress in life, renewal of humanity, and healing the planet will be impossible.

The health science literature emphasizes the moral aspect of personhood as essential to all health issues. The physical, mental, spiritual, and social well-being of individuals involves the moral element of their personhood. This highlights the vital role of the moral self in personhood related to health.

We will explore how scholars perceive the development of the moral self through moral identity and understand the significance of moral identity and the moral self in a person's psychosocial maturity.

Moral Identity of Personhood

The moral aspect of personhood is evident in all human interactions. A person's moral beliefs, feelings, and actions are essential to their true sense of self. Moral identity, in different ways, addresses the question 'Who am I?' and ascribes some level of significance to the answer.

In literature, moral identity is the core psycho-emotional foundation of the moral self. The term moral identity describes a person's fundamental psycho-emotional and behavioral tendencies. The concept of moral identity explains, outlines, and characterizes the psycho-emotional and behavioral patterns of an individual's moral self.

The moral self of a person functions within the framework of moral identity. The underlying psycho-emotional processes of moral identity intricately shape the moral self. The prototype of psycho-emotional and behavioral traits that make up moral identity forms the foundation of the moral self. These traits either promote or hinder prosocial personality development and prosocial tendencies.

Although the moral self carries out all our actions and interactions in the moral realm, they are influenced by one's moral identity. The psycho-emotional processes in a person play a key role when engaging in prosocial and antisocial behaviors, whether acting morally or immorally, causing harm or providing healing to others. This is acknowledged through the moral self of personhood.

The moral identity phenomenon involves the ability to objectify psycho-emotional patterns and behavioral tendencies, and to generalize about these tendencies in a person. This suggests that moral identity can predict how someone will act in moral situations. It helps anticipate how an individual will behave in moral contexts. The psycho-emotional patterns that influence behavior explain both the inconsistency in a person's moral self and the differences among individuals' moral selves.

The prototype psycho-emotional and behavioral traits of a person's moral identity either hinder or promote the development of the individual's moral self. The integration of emotions and thoughts to act and behave in a way that aligns with human nature is essential for the growth of human personhood. Developing personhood involves cultivating moral identity and moral self. It is a lifelong journey of personal growth and self-evolution.

There is only basic awareness of the moral aspect of personhood in childhood. Experts contend that early childhood experiences in the moral domain lay the groundwork for moral identity. The model of one's moral identity develops during childhood; however, moral identity continues to evolve throughout life.

Researchers argue that moral identity does not develop before adolescence and may only exist in a less developed form. They contend that during adolescence, the moral self represents only a basic version of moral identity.[9]

The importance of moral emotion, moral reasoning, and moral

---

[9] Kingsford, J. et.al. The moral self and moral identity: Developmental questions and conceptual challenges. British Journal of Developmental Psychology (Vol.36); 2018

behaviors may or may not be essential to a person's sense of self. Similarly, one's moral identity can be more or less central to one's self-concept. The significance of moral identity to personhood depends on how integral moral human nature is to the individual. Without the moral aspect of personhood, we diminish what truly makes us human. It is our moral nature that sets humans apart from the animal kingdom.

A person's moral identity develops as their sense of personhood integrates moral emotions, thinking, motivation, and behaviors. Usually, it results from following prescribed morals. The calm, integrative, and objective moral identity builds gradually, accumulating over time. It happens throughout a lifetime as a person strives to foster more positive views of their sense of self.

The moral identity forms the foundation of the moral self, which is how people esteem personhood. Perceptions of the moral self, whether aligned or not, are influenced by issues related to moral identity. Researchers have shown that the regenerative design of moral identity, which aims to develop a mature moral self, helps create more aligned and positive perceptions. In moral psychology, regenerative design refers to a mental framework that emphasizes restoring, renewing, and strengthening the moral self of personhood.

Positive views of the moral self originate from a regenerative moral identity that promotes more compassionate thinking, feelings, and actions, as well as the ability to appreciate others in daily life. The renewal of the moral self always aligns with a regenerative moral identity. Designing moral identity in a regenerative way is essential for developing a well-rounded personhood and holistic selfhood.

Moral identity is a flexible aspect of human personality. It can be improved, developed, and renewed to change how the moral self is viewed. The psycho-emotional and behavioral patterns of one's moral identity are adaptable. However, when moral identity becomes fixed and unchangeable, it can lead to moral decline. A rigid moral identity can distort the moral framework of the moral self, negatively affecting the working self-concept and self-identity, which then contributes to moral issues.

The effort to change and improve moral identity requires psychological distancing to evaluate emotional patterns, psychological traits, and behavioral tendencies of one's moral self. The moral self is analyzed to determine whether it supports or hinders overall selfhood and well-being, as well as to promote society's welfare. This process can reveal the positive and negative aspects of moral identity as they affect perceptions of the moral self, which relate to consistency or inconsistency in personhood.

The inherent potential of moral human nature acts as a resource for an individual's moral capacities, which can either be used or left unused in shaping their moral identity. These innate moral capacities, which are fundamental to human nature, tend to be more effective in regenerating moral identity than prescriptive moral norms. The ability of moral human nature to develop moral capacities is connected to the brain's higher cognitive and emotional functions. Specific brain regions and mechanisms are crucial for creating a mature moral self.

Moral identity and the moral self of personhood are linked to human consciousness. Even in its earliest form, human consciousness acts as the gateway to understanding a better way to be human. Both an individual's moral identity and moral self of personhood are shaped by their level of human consciousness. Whether human consciousness is static or evolving, it impacts one's moral identity and moral self in different ways. Higher levels of human consciousness tend to strengthen people's moral identity and moral self more than any moral discipline or legal punishment.

The regenerative design of moral identity, which supports the development of the moral self, is encouraged through self-evolution. People's self-evolution arises from higher levels of human consciousness, with moral consciousness being a vital part of that consciousness. Moral consciousness strengthens the regenerative design of moral identity and aids in developing a mature moral self. When individuals actively pursue self-evolution as a lifelong journey, they also gain a broader view of moral issues, stemming from growth in moral consciousness.

Experientially, the regenerative design of moral identity and the rehabilitation of the moral self mainly result from moral consciousness. Moral consciousness is a subjective feeling, however vague, that one's actions and behaviors lack any known or observable negative moral consequences, even if they are not necessarily the right actions. Moral consciousness helps clarify moral issues during conflicts and dilemmas, aiding in resolving urgent moral questions in daily life. It allows individuals to pursue moral goals without expecting rewards or punishments. As people's moral consciousness develops, so does their mature moral self, continually empowering them to be more effective and relevant in the moral sphere.

Moral consciousness is vital for rebuilding moral identity and developing a mature moral self. It helps reshape the moral self by removing ineffective and harmful psycho-emotional traits, thought patterns, and behavioral tendencies. Its primary focus is on achieving the psychosocial maturity and prosocial tendencies that define a prosocial personality. This process supports the growth of higher-order personhood and psychosocial maturity within the moral domain. Moral consciousness improves perceptions of personhood and promotes the development of a complete selfhood.

The regenerative moral identity is essential for having clear moral goals within a person's sense of self. Moral clarity guides the development of the thinking and behavior patterns of a mature moral self, which are practically shown through psychosocial maturity. Rebuilding moral identity is vital for developing the mature moral self. This mature self benefits not only the individual but also society and humanity. Moreover, the mature moral self strengthens the working self-concept and self-identity. Research indicates that a strong, clear self-concept and well-defined self-identity, as reflected by moral clarity, are crucial for accurate perceptions of oneself and the world.[10]

The static or evolving moral self pertains to the individual's fixed or developing moral identity. The mature moral self depends on the path of the developing moral identity. The regeneration of moral identity presumes a continuous model of moral identity before its development. This view of development indicates that there is an inherent link between the two moral identity constructs in a person, an 'earlier and less mature' version or an 'earlier and more mature' one.

Regarding the development of higher-order personhood and enhancing human life, moral consciousness is crucial. The psychosocial maturity of higher-order personhood, which shapes the mature moral self, is influenced by the regenerative design of moral identity. When people adopt the principles of interdependence and human solidarity, renewing moral identity and rehabilitating the moral self tend to produce better outcomes than strictly following moral systems. The primary purpose of one's moral self is to serve the common good and better humanity, and this is most effectively achieved through cultivating higher-order personhood.

Whether moral, amoral, or immoral, a person's moral identity triggers the behaviors of the moral self. The moral identity underpins one's psycho-emotional processes, moral reasoning, moral sense, and motivations for moral behavior. When someone demonstrates positive psycho-emotional and behavioral tendencies in moral contexts, it reflects the regenerative design of moral identity. This indicates a higher level of moral awareness. It shows that the person's moral clarity remains unaffected by external pressure. There is evidence of an individualized moral self that is not influenced by socially

---

[10] Diehl, M. & Hay E.L. Self-concept differentiation and self-concept clarity across adulthood: Associations with age and psychological well-being. International Journal of Aging and Human Development (Vol. 73), 2011

binding norms.

Some scholars consider moral identity and moral self to be the same, but others argue that moral identity leads to the moral self. The latter group highlights the importance of clearly distinguishing between the concepts of "moral self" and "moral identity." Those who make the distinction see "moral self" and "moral identity" as separate psychological constructs. Even if they are not identical, there is consensus that the moral aspect of personhood greatly influences perceptions of personhood, impacting self-concept, self-identity, and social image.

There is consensus, however, that the psychological and emotional phenomena in question generally align with people's everyday moral sense, reasoning, motivation, and behavioral tendencies. Everyone agrees that moral phenomena form the foundation of moral choices, decisions, and actions that impact people's moral well-being and health, as well as society's welfare. These phenomena also emphasize that a person's moral self is connected to their moral health and that moral health is a vital part of overall health.

The idea of moral identity has gained increasing attention in social and developmental psychology.[11] Health experts and researchers highlight that moral identity is crucial for human maturity and self-awareness. It plays a role in developing a mature moral self, psychosocial growth, and a person's moral well-being. It influences all areas of life, including health, relationships, and every aspect of our human experience.

Integrating a high level of moral awareness into one's self-awareness shapes the psychological and emotional processes involved in the regenerative design of moral identity, which repairs and renews a person's moral self. The literature indicates that people's moral identity can change for better or worse

---

[11] Hardy, S. A., & Carlo, G. Moral identity: What is it, how does it develop, and is it linked to moral action? Society for Research in Child Development; 2011.

over their lifetime.

Moral Self: The Core of Personhood

The "moral self" is the highest level of a person's self-identity. The term "moral self" is typically used to emphasize the everyday patterns of moral feelings, reasoning, and behavioral tendencies that comprise a person's moral identity, including both explicit and implicit elements. In literature, the term "moral self" describes how we perceive ourselves and others morally, reflected in our thoughts, feelings, actions, and behaviors.

Socio-cultural anthropologists consider the moral self to be the core of personhood.[12] Among humanists, the moral self in personhood is described as a collection of moral emotions and behaviors that demonstrate an individual's moral abilities and define what it means to be human.[13]

From a psychosocial perspective, the moral self of personhood influences how individuals see themselves and how others see them. It provides the perceptual basis for evaluating oneself and understanding others' perceptions. The moral self serves as the overall principle that encompasses personhood, specifically concerning a person's self-awareness. It is always crucial to perceptions of personhood and plays a key role in developing self-concept and self-identity. It directly affects a person's social image. The integrity of a moral self's consistent, purposeful nature is vital for maintaining personhood and emotional stability.

The moral self profoundly influences how a person functions in all areas of life. It motivates us to engage constantly and proactively with various responsibilities to ourselves and others. The moral self of personhood defines what it means to be human and how one relates to oneself and others. The insightful understanding of one's moral self shows how one is being human in

---

[12] Hardy, S. A., & Carlo, G. Moral identity: What is it, how does it develop, and is it linked to moral action? Society for Research in Child Development; 2011.
[13] Copson A, Donnellan L, Norman R. Understanding Humanism. Routledge, 2023

society.

The moral self of personhood allows individuals to take on multiple responsibilities, work toward the common good, and promote human solidarity. An individual's moral self reveals the psycho-emotional aspects of personhood that influence or hinder positive human traits. In all relationships, the moral self affects a person's psychosocial maturity. The development and expression of one's psychosocial maturity happen through a mature moral self.

Health literature considers the moral self essential in healthcare. Modern science shows that people who maintain strong moral standards are much less likely to face physical, mental, and social health issues.[14] The moral self affects whether we feel balanced and at peace or out of sorts. Whether someone feels settled and consistent or unsettled and mainly inconsistent depends on their moral self.

The moral self of personhood affects not only all aspects of human health but also the future of humanity. Society's well-being and the fate of humankind are deeply connected to the influence of the moral self in life. The moral self can either promote or hinder the welfare of society and humanity. A mature moral self is crucial for creating a healthier society and a better future for humankind.

In the postmodern world, we often overlook the influence of the moral self on personhood. We often overlook how it influences our daily thoughts and actions. We rarely consider how the moral self impacts ourselves and others. Evidence from life shows that a mature moral self is desperately needed in the postmodern world to improve human life in all its aspects.

The moral self highlights the agentic moral abilities of an autonomous and interdependent individual. Essentially, human moral capacities are centered

---

[14] Weziah-Bailowolska, D. et.al. Prospective associations between strengths of moral character and health: longitudinal evidence from survey and insurance claims data Social Psychiatry and Psychiatry Epidemiology (Vol. 58); 2023.

on doing good, avoiding harm, and developing a sense of otherness. The moral self functions as a self-regulating system of personhood, primarily guided by emotional signals and stored as procedural knowledge. In this context, procedural knowledge refers to the "know-how" or fundamental moral skill needed to perform moral tasks and fulfill obligations. This frames the moral self within the prototype psycho-emotional traits that define a person's moral identity. It underscores that the behavioral structure of the moral self is rooted in one's moral identity.

The extent to which someone develops their moral self is supported by renewing their moral identity. An individual's moral identity and moral self can follow the paths of moral conscience or moral awareness. Essentially, the idea of the moral self in personhood relates to the moral duty to respect the fundamental human dignity of everyone. Evidence from life shows us that this process happens more effectively through moral awareness. The moral abilities that demonstrate refined and heightened moral sensitivity are influenced by moral awareness.

The moral self of personhood is essential to how we see others and how they see us. Perceptions of personhood develop through the interaction of psychological, emotional, and behavioral patterns. Our thoughts, feelings, and actions in the moral realm shape how we view each other's moral selves.

The moral self always influences how we view ourselves as individuals. Usually, our understanding of what it means to be human, both to ourselves and others, develops through the functioning of the moral self. Our perceptions of who we are and how others see us are primarily based on observable psycho-emotional and behavioral patterns. The perceptions of the moral self indicate whether our sense of personhood is consistent or inconsistent.

Researchers highlight that the moral self is a dynamic part of personhood shaped by our perceptions of ourselves and others.[15] The moral self is essential in how we view ourselves and how others see us. Positive views of one's personhood are influenced mainly by a prosocial personality, especially when psycho-emotional patterns and behavioral tendencies drive relevant positive actions and prosocial inclinations.

The effort we invest in developing the moral self shows how vital the moral self is to one's sense of personhood. Perceptions of personhood are essential to self-concept, self-identity, and social image. They also play a key role in self-esteem, well-being, and health. When the moral self guides behaviors to balance self-interest with the needs of others, it promotes positive perceptions of personhood.

Self-concept, self-identity, and social image all stem from how we perceive an individual's personhood. How we view the moral self can either strengthen or weaken our everyday self-concept and self-identity. These aspects are adaptable and vary depending on the context, mirroring a person's perception of their personhood. Moreover, perceptions of the moral self influence social image, which can be either positive or negative.

Consistency is the primary concern when it comes to one's personhood. Experts say that everyday thoughts, feelings, and behaviors come from a motivation to keep the consistency of personhood.[16] This need for consistency is crucial for health, well-being, and happiness. The psychological desire for consistency depends on how we and others see us. Personhood consistency mainly depends on perceptions of the moral self within personhood.

When consistency of personhood is important, perceptions related to

---

[15] Christner, N. et. al. Emotion understanding and the moral self-concept as motivators of prosocial behavior in middle childhood. Journal of Cognitive Development; July-September, 2020

[16] Merenda, P. Similarities between Prescott Lecky's Theory of Self-Consistency and Carl Rogers' Self-Theory. Psychological Reports (Vol. 107); 2010

the moral aspect of someone's personhood become even more significant than physical and mental perceptions. The perceptions of the moral self have the most significant impact on maintaining the consistency of personhood. A holistic individual strives to cultivate and uphold positive perceptions by developing the moral self to preserve the integrity of personhood.

The consistency of personhood depends on how the moral self is viewed within a person's working self-concept and self-identity. Whether the moral identity is fixed or evolving affects perceptions of the moral self, which in turn influences whether personhood stays consistent. Keeping alignment between the individual's moral identity and moral self—reflected in their working self-concept, self-identity, and social image—is crucial for maintaining stable personhood.

The moral self of a person plays a crucial role in how one perceives their working self-concept and self-identity. The moral self of personhood is vital to the working self-concept and self-identity, as well as to a person's social image. Our perceptions of who we are to ourselves and others are based on the working self-concept and self-identity.

The perception of the moral self is central to a person's working self-concept and self-identity. We understand and evaluate personhood based on how we perceive others' working self-concept and self-identity. The strength, honesty, character, and psychosocial maturity of higher-level personhood are reflected through a person's working self-concept and self-identity.

The working self-concept and self-identity are crucial to a person's social image and self-esteem. A person's social image and self-esteem are influenced either positively or negatively by their moral self's behaviors. The working self-concept and self-identity can help shape and improve emotional patterns, psychological traits, and behavioral tendencies of the moral self, which in turn have a positive impact on social image and self-esteem.

The positive and negative effects we experience daily from others' actions mainly reflect their moral character. These behaviors reveal whether someone has a developing, mature, or weak and rigid moral self. Either type shapes a person's psychosocial maturity. The chaotic and turbulent world we live in indicates a serious problem of disordered personhood, leading to behaviors driven by self-disintegration. People's actions do not necessarily reveal the level of higher-order psychosocial maturity.

People's moral self can either be evolving and maturing or static, rigid, weak, and malignant. The successful cultivation of society's moral health should focus on people's self-evolution and higher-order personhood rather than merely developing the mental abilities to comply with and conform to moral rules. Society needs to prioritize the mature moral self, which is cultivated through moral consciousness. The focus on traditional morality's ideals and norms shifts attention away from self-evolution and psychosocial maturity.

The moral self primarily focuses on addressing pressing moral dilemmas and upholding moral norms and standards. People exhibit strong moral motivation to tackle moral challenges and problems when moral awareness is a key part of the moral self.

Today, we examine cultural factors and influences that dangerously weaken the integrity of personhood and holistic self-awareness. We confront the harmful moral self that corrupts both identity and self-concept. The struggle with people's problematic working self-image and self-identity reflects a weaker experience of consistent personhood. The desire to maintain a stable and positive social image shows efforts to hide self-disintegration. We cope with life by enduring a chaotic, disorderly sense of self and an illusion of stability.

As social, environmental, technological, and economic conditions evolve, people's moral selves continuously face challenges in adapting to various socio-cultural phenomena and finding new solutions. Recognizing one's moral self serves as a way to evaluate our lifestyles and ways of living in modern society, and to explore ways to improve the quality of human life for everyone. The development of the moral self is a pathway to adjusting to new ways of living in the world.

The development of a person's moral self usually advances very slowly. This is especially true for those who feel limited by strict thinking, values, and attitudes in an environment of social and cultural change. However, the improvements in humane qualities of the mature moral self within one's self-concept and self-identity are valuable. These positive views of personhood enhance well-being, overall health, and society's welfare.

The mature moral self of each individual can serve as a guide to others regarding the importance of consistency in character, a holistic sense of self, and the psychosocial maturity required in our society. There is always the potential for one's moral identity and moral self to reflect either the traits and qualities of moral exemplars or the typical features of a conventional moral person.

When a person's moral self attributes explicitly align with the moral identity and moral self of a moral exemplar, there is less emphasis on obedience and behavioral conformity to moral standards and more focus on self-growth and psychosocial maturity—the individual acts with moral responsibility that surpasses what is required by normative morality. There is no fixed moral self tied to any rigid moral system for the working self-concept or self-identity, but only the dynamic processes of personal development.

Although researchers recognize that individual differences in a person's moral self stem from various perspectives, they lack clarity on what defines the core of the moral self.[17] While they have a better understanding of moral thought and behavior, current research only provides an integrated framework related to the concept of the moral self in personhood. Scholars argue that the challenge for researchers is to determine how the moral self develops.

---

[17] Zhu, W. et al. Neural correlates of individual differences in moral identity and its positive moral function. Journal of Neuropsychology; May 2024

The Static vs. Evolving Moral Self

One's personhood being relational by nature emphasizes that the moral self is primarily connected to all the relationships we form and maintain. In the moral realm, the framework of relationship patterns is rooted in the moral self. The moral self of personhood functions as the main resource for making decisions about how to perceive, understand, and act humanely. A mature moral self highly values all human relationships, without expectations or judgments.

The role of the moral self has attracted significant theoretical and empirical interest in recent decades. A person's moral self is considered crucial in shaping worldviews, which can either enhance or harm their life. The moral aspects of personality style and function are seen as key to revealing the hidden moral identity linked to the moral self, indicating whether individuals are human or inhuman. Greater focus is placed on moral identity to understand how people's daily psychological, emotional, and behavioral patterns are influenced by their moral selves.

Typically, people develop their moral self by adopting a set of moral values. This process begins in early childhood through socialization, which is connected to their society's moral culture. The moral culture, grounded in a universal set of moral ideals and principles, supports the socialization process. Society's moral culture includes interdisciplinary abstract norms mainly aimed at the shared understanding of what is good, right, and just.

The main goal of the socialization process is to prepare an individual to be a responsible member of society by developing a moral self. Childhood upbringing focuses on instilling moral thinking, feelings, and behaviors that last a lifetime. It involves the overall psycho-emotional-social development of personhood to shape the values and actions of the moral self. The basic form of the moral self during childhood lays the foundation for the growth of the moral self. This may or may not occur throughout a person's lifetime.

Early childhood experiences in the moral domain lay the foundation of the moral self. There are two other important factors to consider when exploring the origin of the moral self. First, an individual's moral identity is closely linked to their personal history, nationality, ethnicity, religion, and the social and cultural context of their time. Sociocultural and historical influences strongly shape a person's self-identity and significantly affect their typical psycho-emotional and behavioral traits related to moral identity. Additionally, different cultures express and emphasize an individual's moral self in various ways within the moral domain. Because everyone's moral self is rooted in unique sociocultural and historical backgrounds, it varies across society, culture, and history.

Typically, a person's moral self is centered on the moral standards of society's culture. It is a socially binding moral identity that relies on bureaucratic moral rationality and truth. Social institutions such as family, religion, law, and education shape this moral self. The socially binding moral self is linked with moral ideals and principles embedded in social institutions. It influences daily values, attitudes, beliefs, and behaviors. The moral framework behind people's everyday actions is based on institutional rationality and truth. Social institutions aim to develop the moral self in individuals to encourage prosocial personalities and behaviors. This same moral self often affects society's social, economic, and political policies at both national and international levels. However, the relevance and effectiveness of the socially binding moral self in addressing urgent moral dilemmas and challenges remain subject to debate.

When confronted with moral complexities, the socially binding moral self is limited by boundaries. It tends to focus on abstract moral principles and ideals that are disconnected from urgent moral issues of the present, leading to everyday moral dilemmas and conflicts. It is often constrained by rules and norms that are irrelevant or outdated regarding pressing moral concerns.

Life experiences show that the moral complexities in any present moment are not always within what the socially accepted moral self considers enough. As often seen in the moral realm, the range of problems, issues, and challenges is endless. They go beyond the limits of traditional morality and other human control systems.

Usually, the pursuit of traditional morality mainly aims to be perceived as a decent person and/or to show that one is either blameless or blameworthy in moral matters. However, if being a moral person is limited to focusing on maintaining a moral self to meet social expectations, it can weaken the moral self needed to address more urgent moral problems and dilemmas beyond the scope of conventional morality. Traditional morality and society's moral culture often hinder the development of the mature moral self necessary in today's world.

When individuals rely on society's moral culture to shape their moral self, their moral identity aligns with the accepted moral views of that society. This moral self shows tendencies toward different behaviors through denial of objective truth and self-deception. The moral perspectives of social institutions cause people to experience moral self-dissonance. This often manifests in their struggles with issues of integrity, character, and psychosocial maturity.

We encounter people every day who, while immersed in conventional morality, exhibit a moral self involved in unconscionable behaviors, nefarious activities, and viciousness. When the moral self aligns with a society's moral culture, it more easily finds opportunities to develop deviant and malicious tendencies. Evidence from life clearly shows that the moral self, consistent with society's moral worldviews, is becoming increasingly ineffective at addressing modern moral dilemmas and conflicts.

Additionally, we know that in daily life, there are competing motivations that lead people to act in ways different from the moral rules guiding their moral self. People often find themselves either under social or cultural pressure to respond a certain way or confused about why they do what they do. It is common for us to be indifferent to the harmful effects and consequences of evil actions that conflict with the socially binding moral self.

The moral self predicts whether moral reasoning and motivation will be competent or incompetent when facing moral challenges and problems in the postmodern world. The highly effective moral self in the postmodern moral realm is built on a moral aptitude that is not limited by moral ideals that define who is moral and how one acts morally.

Being a moral person today isn't just about maintaining human decency and harmony. Moreover, human decency goes beyond simple social politeness and pleasantries, which often hide a malicious moral self. Furthermore, true harmony in human life isn't about ignoring urgent moral issues that require more empathetic understanding and a sense of connection to our shared humanity.

In a changing and complex moral landscape, the moral self must help us respond effectively, relevantly, and positively to evolving social and cultural circumstances. We need the moral ability that functions well in new life situations. Empathetic humanity isn't just about prosocial behaviors and avoiding antisocial acts but about tackling urgent moral issues and dilemmas that undermine interdependence, human solidarity, and our connection to the web of life.

In a world transformed into a global village, the ability of the moral self to promote social integration and cohesion requires more than traditional morality and abstract principles. It is evident that interdependence and human solidarity are urgent issues in today's moral landscape. Common human concerns in the postmodern era are poorly and ineffectively addressed by the moral self rooted in traditional morality. Life experiences show that, in our times, there are situations, issues, and events in the moral realm where we respond ineffectively with the binding moral self. The socially binding moral self in postmodern times cannot develop moral awareness quickly enough to meet moral demands. When the rigid and undeveloped moral self limits people's moral reasoning and motivation, the nuanced reasoning of the moral self across the moral domain diminishes.

In the moral realm, people should prioritize the purpose and motivation behind the common good over self-interest and personal preferences. The subtle understanding of objective existential truth by the moral self in modern times relies on moral consciousness. With moral consciousness, we become more in tune with the moral nature of the present moment and are less likely to get caught up in moral standards, conflicts, or dilemmas. We respond to moral issues by recognizing the objective truth within the moral domain.

Scholars explain that, unlike the binding moral self, there can be an individualizing moral self. This moral self reflects the development of cognitive, psycho-emotional, and psychosocial aspects within a person. It does not overlap with the self shaped by socio-cultural and historical contexts. The individualizing moral self develops through the regenerative process of moral identity influenced by evolving moral consciousness.

A person's moral consciousness enhances moral awareness and clarity about pressing moral issues and entities. The processes of attention, perception, and interpretation of moral topics primarily stem from one's moral consciousness. In everyday life, conventional morality establishes mental and emotional boundaries for individuals' moral selves. The deeper moral awareness, which forms broad views within the moral domain, originates from moral consciousness rather than moral conscience. This profound moral awareness sets the binding moral self apart from the more mature, individualizing moral self.

The individualizing moral self is essential for a person's ability to act morally effectively in postmodern times. When dealing with moral issues, moral consciousness forms the mental and behavioral mechanisms of the moral self, distinct from those created by the socially binding moral self. Through moral consciousness, the individualizing moral self can detach from the socially binding moral self.

The corrupt and misguided moral identity that permits harm to others reemerges through the process of personalizing the moral self. This identity reflects the individual's priorities, values, and goals, and is not solely grounded in institutional or cultural moral reasoning. Moral consciousness acts as the pathway to restore one's moral identity and heal the moral self.

The moral awareness of an individual shapes the developed moral self. This developed self shows the ability to think, feel, and act in ways that go beyond traditional morality. It is not limited by institutional reasoning or bureaucratic truths. Instead, it pushes back against moral boundaries created by society's moral culture, challenging or expanding moral responses.

This represents the moral self of personhood that authentically reacts to pressing moral issues, even if the response diverges from traditional morality's standards, beliefs, or values. The mature moral self cultivates psychosocial maturity, helping individuals more effectively confront and resolve moral dilemmas. Its responses are always pertinent to the moral entity, regardless of social disapproval or punishment.

The mature moral self is defined by a mindset of someone working to renew their moral identity. The static moral self comes from indifference toward a corrupt and degenerate moral identity. In a fast-changing world, an unchallenged moral identity often appears in people as a rigid, weak, and degraded moral self.

The regenerative process of moral identity occurs when people consistently pursue higher levels of personhood, which are reflected in their personal integrity, character, resilience, and psychosocial maturity as a fully developed moral self. It is through regenerating moral identity and restoring the moral self that we grow and enrich our sense of self, positively impacting society's well-being.

In our current era, the failure of traditional morality and abstract theories of morality and human control systems has led researchers to explore the psychological concept of moral identity and moral self. Research evidence shows that the moral self, which influences one's health and humanity, aligns with the moral drive—the resource called moral identity—within individuals' psycho-emotional processes, thought patterns, and behavioral tendencies.[18]

The moral conflicts, issues, and dilemmas that negatively influence people's moral responses and responsibilities can also promote the renewal of their moral identity and foster the development of a mature moral self. In a world filled with moral uncertainties, we must continuously evaluate and develop our moral identity through self-reflection to create an individualized moral self. A renewing moral identity is crucial for restoring the moral self. A key aspect of shaping an individual's moral self is the ability to perform objective and independent self-assessments. This process happens constantly in daily life as life unfolds in the present and is driven by moral awareness. Moral awareness underpins people's tendency to understand who they truly are, what they genuinely stand for, and how much value they assign to human life.

The individualizing moral self supports moral reasoning and the ability to recognize the many different shades of gray that emerge in a world of human progress, scientific determinism, and technological inventions. It comes from the understanding that a black-and-white view of traditional morality causes many unavoidable problems, such as war, genocide, terrorism, violations of fundamental human rights, and everyday issues like crime, domestic violence, suicide, homicide, and other wrongdoings. Developing people's mature moral selves is essential for psychosocial maturity in the postmodern world to

---

[18] Blasi, A. The development of identity: Some implications for moral functioning. In G. G. Noam & T. E. Wren (Eds.) The moral self. MIT Press; 1993.

effectively tackle social challenges and issues.

The individualizing moral self gives people a life orientation that goes beyond traditional or cultural morality. It helps break free from thinking patterns that exclude and marginalize others, which weaken social bonds. Instead, it redirects individuals toward others and encourages thinking based on interdependence, human solidarity, and the common good. Through moral awareness, the individualizing moral self creates a more meaningful, purposeful, and effective moral framework, shaping the thoughts, feelings, and behaviors of the mature moral self.

The individualizing moral self effectively resolves moral conflicts and overcomes dilemmas. It demonstrates, to oneself and others, a tendency toward prosocial traits and behaviors. It emphasizes humaneness, empathetic friendliness, altruism, and higher life goals, rather than focusing on moral rules and principles. Usually, this is not highlighted by one's socially binding moral self, which is guided by conventional morality.

The individualizing moral self mainly develops through people cultivating advanced personhood. The mature moral self and psychosocial maturity result from higher-level personhood and are vital in today's society. This means we must dedicate ourselves to lifelong self-improvement and foster moral awareness. Moral consciousness, which encourages higher-level personhood, arises from self-evolution. It establishes the foundation for the proper criteria used to distinguish truly moral behavior from other positive behaviors seen in both humans and non-humans.

Moral consciousness at each moment in the moral realm triggers the reflective evaluation of the individualizing moral self. This self develops through real-life experiences rather than by following abstract societal ideals of morality. While norms serve as standards, patterns, rules, and guidelines for expected behaviors, they also define the boundaries and limitations of moral reasoning and motivation. The individualizing moral self embodies the mature moral self, representing higher-order personhood through people's psychosocial development.

The most vital tool for fostering higher-order personhood is moral consciousness. This stems from neurobiology rather than culture. The best explanation of higher-order personhood involves multiple brain functions that enhance the development of moral identity and moral self. These neurological processes enable individuals to reach their full moral potential in life. The natural course of meaningful human transformation relies on the innate mechanisms of the human brain that support the growth of a mature moral self and psychosocial maturity. A person's neurobiological state is essential for developing a complete self, overall health, and a more compassionate society.

The human species evolved to be moral beings through natural selection. The development of higher cognitive and emotional abilities related to morality was made possible by human evolution and the moral nature of humanity. The subsequent psychological and cultural evolution of human society led to the creation of systems of morality, which started to define what it means to be a moral self. Social and cultural changes have enabled humans to develop moral standards for acceptable behavior, which are now used to describe a person's moral identity. This shows that the socially binding moral self is rooted in human culture, while the individualizing moral self arises from the innate moral capacities of an individual.

The moral environment of a society reflects the moral character of its people. This moral character is a key indicator and vital part of society's well-being, resilience, and stability. The moral health of society comes from individuals, not from moral ideals embedded in social institutions, legal systems, or culture. When harmful and dangerous behaviors go unnoticed—which often happens in today's world—that signals a static moral character. Improving the moral environment of society depends on each person continually working to renew their moral identity and restore their moral self.

A society functions well when its members possess a mature moral self. However, today's societal moral climate often suggests that an individual's moral self is seen as incompatible with concepts like otherness, interdependence, human solidarity, and coexistence. It does not effectively promote thoughts and actions that enhance moral well-being. This moral environment isn't the result of a lack of standards or moral guidelines but rather due to underdeveloped moral awareness. In a constantly changing world, appropriate and effective moral responses are shaped more by moral awareness than by fixed moral ideals or social, cultural, and historical contexts. Therefore, the moral self must be future-focused and adaptable, rather than stuck in outdated habits. True altruism, other-centered thinking, interdependence, solidarity, and meaningful coexistence come from a moral self rooted in higher-order personhood, distinct from one that merely obeys external moral pressures.

The moral self involves more than just having prosocial intentions. If the moral self is simply defined as an awareness of "human decency" – doing no harm or being right and just – then it can reasonably be understood through social interactions. However, if it is defined as the internalization of emotional and behavioral standards within personhood, then it depends on the individualizing moral self. More than the binding moral self, the individualizing moral self of people makes a richer contribution to improving the moral environment in the world. People's higher-order personhood is a prerequisite for the mature moral self and psychosocial maturity, which are necessary to change the moral landscape in today's world.

POSTMODERN WORLD IMPACT ON MORAL SELF

This is a challenging and demanding time in human history. We live in a world filled with geopolitical tensions and worldwide instability. The political, economic, cultural, and social uncertainties are profoundly impacting the lives of ordinary people. Unlike previous eras, we are charting unknown waters of moral chaos. We are overwhelmed by moral conflicts, dilemmas, and uncertainties.

We live in a world of intense conflicts among rival groups and nations. These conflicts seriously threaten humanity's future. Modern science and technology have vastly improved human life, but have also enabled modern warfare. Many conflicts worldwide are driven by biological, chemical, and nuclear weapons, which not only destroy nations but also threaten humanity's survival and the planet's future.

We live in a world where modern warfare is unlike anything previous generations have experienced. Every day, we see disturbing war horrors broadcast live on television and social media, revealing human brutality. Modern weaponry presents an existential threat of catastrophic scale. The risk of planetary destruction is no longer just science fiction or a distant threat. The looming danger of disaster causes everyone to feel a sense of existential anxiety in our world.

We live in a world overwhelmed by existential angst, which negatively affects the human mind both individually and collectively. This existential dread disrupts the daily routines and activities of ordinary people, making it hard for them to find joy in small things. Everyone understands that it's one thing when angry people are armed with fists and sticks, but quite another when psychopathic political leaders are leading an army using military machinery in warfare. Many wise scholars and ordinary citizens debate whether the future of humanity hangs by a thin thread. No one will deny that, in the postmodern world, the greatest threat to humanity's survival is humanly depraved world leaders.

We live in a world filled with dictators, tyrants, despots, fascists, totalitarian regimes, and religious, political, and ideological fanatics. Their rhetorical threats and vicious actions contribute to widespread anxiety among people. The moral corruption of many modern politicians, heads of state, and religious leaders negatively affects the mental health of people in many countries. Additionally, we live in a world controlled by a small group of oligarchs and tycoons. Their self-interest and ambitions drive geopolitical conflicts with severe consequences. In managing the "business" of the world, they reveal their unruly moral character. Their lifestyles and behaviors show total depravity and a complete disregard for humanity.

However, it is not only malicious political leaders, regimes, unscrupulous religious leaders, or business tycoons who threaten humanity. We live in a world where people generally go about their daily lives without even considering the risk of an unprecedented, catastrophic event unfolding through our everyday actions. We underestimate the ripple effects of modern dreams, ambitions, and relentless material greed on the survival of our planet. We never see it as a problem that our insatiable desires deny basic survival needs to a large portion of humanity. The generations of our time pursue life goals, priorities, and lifestyles that ignore the serious consequences that individual and collective actions can have on humanity's future.

Often, we avoid thinking about the potentially disastrous consequences of our modern scientific and technological pursuits. Most of us remain unaware of or deny the real risk of an irreversible catastrophe for humanity and the planet, caused by greed, neglect, environmental abuse, and interference with nature and the universe. Every day, ecologists, environmentalists, social activists, cultural critics, interdisciplinary experts, and philanthropists warn about its likelihood, but it seems to fall on deaf ears.

Today, around the world, evil acts remain an endless plague. Incidents of brutal, heinous, and vicious crimes in society are at record levels and becoming uncontrollable. Society's moral fabric seems unable to stop blatant corruption, illegal abuse of power, and malicious exploitation of society's most vulnerable members. Society's morality and laws fail to prevent ongoing criminal behavior, felonious activities, and evil deeds that happen constantly.

Like past generations, we depend on prescriptive and normative morality to shape our moral identity. However, life experience shows that traditional morality is becoming less effective in the changing moral landscape of postmodern times. Our way of living in modern society demonstrates indifference and neglect toward the moral core of individual personhood. More people tend to think, feel, and act in ways that go against what it means to be human. The disturbing number of brutal deaths in war, violent homicides, and mass suicides reveals inhumanity within society. No moral tradition, legal system, or moral goal seems to make a difference in improving the declining moral environment of modern society.

Amidst the moral chaos in an unstable world, the rapid growth of scientific innovation, technology, and globalization has a profound impact on human life, affecting it both positively and negatively. While we focus on the benefits, we often overlook the adverse effects that profoundly impact what it means to be human. Today, the human individual is frequently viewed as an automaton, lacking the essential qualities of metaphysical human nature.

In modern society, we relate to people who behave no differently than robots. Robotic humans exemplify a type of character that is soulless, cold-hearted, and unfeeling. Without human empathy, sensitivity, and compassion, people's destructive tendencies now rival the destructive power of war machinery. Individuals destroy and ravage each other without fear, remorse, or guilt. The widespread existence of cruelty and inhumane treatment of fellow humans in society reveals everyday human depravity and the decline of moral values.

The concept of "human progress" in postmodern times has also influenced a complex human reality. Technologization, secularization, and rationalization of the modern world have resulted in a "new" human phenomenon. Experts contend that widespread societal changes accompany the emergence of the "new" human reality. They recognize both the positive and negative impacts of the "new" human phenomenon in the postmodern world.

The positives mainly involve more people in the postmodern world developing a new human consciousness. It is experienced through human interactions based on principles of empathetic friendliness, interdependence, and human solidarity. They acknowledge objective truth, respect cultural differences, and cultivate multicultural thinking. On a social level, this new human consciousness is visible in people intentionally working to develop global perspectives and pursue reforms focused on racial justice and equality.

However, the negatives are revealed by the unchecked power of large corporations, oligarchs, business moguls, and tech tycoons, along with widespread misinformation, privacy erosion, and the widening gap between the haves and the have-nots. The diverse personality styles, non-traditional understandings of gender identity and roles, and unorthodox sexual attractions and gratifications also demonstrate the negative consequences. The "new" human phenomenon presents numerous moral challenges and problems unique to our times.

The "new" human reality is shaping psycho-emotional processes that influence daily behaviors. The "new" human phenomenon shows that the demands on people's moral selves conflict with traditional moral reasoning and motivations for actions. On a personal level, this has created many uncertainties about one's sense of personhood and selfhood. As hard as it may be to accept, we are at odds with ourselves and feel insecure in our skin in today's society. In daily life, the moral self that people claim reveals an unstable personhood and a fluid sense of identity.

On the societal level, the "new" human phenomenon is shaping how people behave at home, in their communities, and around the world. Evidence shows that we are becoming less able to treat others the way we want to be treated. Our way of being human is negatively affecting relationship patterns and breaking social norms. The insensitive and inhumane treatment of others highlights human decline in today's world. The hoaxes, fraudsters, tricksters, con artists, 'black hats,' and similar individuals have become comfortable and confident in their actions, despite the harm they cause. In modern society, the moral self connected to the "new" human phenomenon is actively influencing the direction of human life.

Some cultural critics argue that the "new" human reality worsens the moral challenges faced by people in modern society. People struggle to understand and recognize what is genuinely human in others. In a constantly changing world, they are overwhelmed by moral uncertainties. These uncertainties weaken their sense of self-consistency and coherence. Moral dilemmas cause them to think and act in ways that undermine their sense of self. Some suggest this is because people survive with a moral self shaped by conventional morality. When faced with urgent moral issues in daily life, their fragile, flawed, and rigid moral selves fail to guide them effectively.

The global culture of our era is unlike any other in human history. Driven by materialism, consumerism, individualism, and hedonism, it is undeniably the dominant force in the post-modern world. These "isms" shape our dreams and ambitions for self-fulfillment, many of which reflect the influence of a harmful moral self. They help define the prevailing global moral framework. This is evident in the widespread presence of pathological self-centeredness and utilitarian individualism. The negative impact of cultural factors on the moral self leads to harmful behaviors and numerous adverse consequences for moral health, both personally and collectively.

Modernity has brought significant changes to what it means to be human today. On one hand, the postmodern world offers unparalleled opportunities for human growth and progress; on the other hand, it presents unprecedented and unique challenges to our understanding of humanity. There is no clear certainty about what truly matters in moral terms, and people often feel unsure when facing moral dilemmas, conflicts, challenges, and struggles. The global moral landscape suggests that traditional morality might hinder individuals' moral development, preventing it from becoming a means to create a better way to be human. Amidst all the scientific rationalism and comfort of modern life, many people slip into barbaric behaviors.

In today's moral landscape, traditional boundaries and constraints of morality impair the effectiveness of the moral self. The moral reasoning based on outdated ideals and principles causes people to judge and condemn quickly, and it also makes them less capable of demonstrating empathy, mutuality, and tolerance. It weakens the psychosocial maturity needed for appropriate behavior in a rapidly changing world. People operate with a moral self that is ineffective at self-regulation, acting responsibly, and addressing urgent moral issues. The moral self, which is relevant to our times, does not receive the attention it deserves. We fail to meet the higher demands of personhood necessary for psychosocial maturity—thinking, feeling, and being human. Self-evolution is not prioritized, and we do not develop higher-level personhood.

In today's way of thinking and living, there is, on one hand, too much certainty about the moral self of personhood, which leads people to assert themselves; on the other hand, there is too much moral confusion in the world. Life experience shows that people's problematic moral self isn't the disoriented one but the one that exhibits rigid, uncompromising, and unwavering moral convictions.

Throughout recorded history, people have lamented the decline of kindness, honesty, cooperation, civility, and decency. But today, voices of concerned individuals worldwide echo deep worries that this decline in society's moral health is not only harming public well-being but also threatening human existence. The perceived decline in moral health among modern people, despite any signs of improvement, suggests that the malignant moral self within individuals is worsening, possibly becoming irremediable like terminal cancer.

We see this in public leaders who, stemming from a rigid, weak, and corrupt moral self, commit horrible, disgusting, and heinous acts on the world stage. It has encouraged some unscrupulous world leaders even to justify ethnic cleansing and genocide. Loathsome and despicable politicians and religious leaders pretend to be moral authorities with their twisted, corrupt, and evil moral selves. We know of oligarchs, tycoons, and moguls building empires based on wealth gained by crushing the lives of the poor masses. We live in a world where politicians, oligarchs, tycoons, and religious leaders evade the consequences of their evil actions, affecting the daily lives of millions.

There is certainly no shortage of serious problems in the world caused by people's moral selves. Besides the more obvious violent outcomes of wars, political oppression, global and domestic terrorism, social violence, and heinous crimes seen on TV, there are more localized concerns about community and national socio-economic-political issues affecting daily life. We have become accustomed to hearing about, and even knowing, people who can no longer live normal daily lives, such as owning a home, falling in love, getting married, raising a family, denying healthcare when sick, and blocking the right to die with dignity.

Are we collectively worsening the global health crisis of moral decline to our own destruction? Do all the current evils in the modern world indicate that the moral core of personhood is dead today?

We will evaluate the impact of postmodernity on the moral self from four contemporary viewpoints: (1) human culture, (2) human self-identity, (3) human health, and (4) human value.

Contemporary Human Culture

No one can escape the harmful influence of cultural factors that distort the moral foundation of life. Constant material cravings, the pursuit of pleasure, and salacious desires hinder one's pursuit of higher ideals and purposes. This is clear not only in the widespread presence of evil in our world but also in daily self-deceptions, denials, blame-shifting, malicious intentions, and many other problematic patterns of thought and behavior.

The subtle influence of global culture on the moral self often goes unnoticed in people's daily lives. Usually, there is a moral outlook that aligns with cultural values and attitudes. This stems from a static, rigid, and undeveloped moral self, which has caused individuals to be mostly self-focused when considering life's meaning, purpose, values, priorities, and goals.

Today, we enjoy more comfortable lifestyles in informed environments and benefit from advancements in science and technology. We increase in knowledge, wealth, and prosperity while pursuing the "good life." However, evidence also shows that as people become obsessed with wealth, elitism, and hedonistic desires, they tend to overlook the problems, both obvious and hidden, that the moral self creates for themselves and others.

Despite material wealth and modern luxuries, people often feel an underlying emptiness and a lack of purpose in life. This has driven an unstoppable desire to "feel good" and steer clear of anything painful. The "feel good" culture today, regardless of whether actions are right or wrong, is backed by our reliance on "quick fixes" in society. In this setting, we accept a moral self that tolerates addictions, misuse of prescription drugs and hallucinogens, acting on impulses, engaging in destructive behaviors, and much more.

Many of the "quick-fix" solutions in our society directly contribute to a corrupted moral environment. These "quick-fix" solutions often benefit dishonest and corrupt individuals through secretive, behind-closed-doors deals, subjugate the powerless and marginalized members of society, promote malicious practices for personal gain, exploit public office for selfish reasons, and more.

People often cling to "quick-fix" solutions instead of tackling the root causes of modern problems, whether personal or societal. When we embrace the "feel good" culture and chase after "quick fixes," we ignore the importance of the moral self. Without paying attention to the moral self, which influences our everyday actions, many social, global, and health issues remain unresolved or are poorly managed.

In the postmodern world, the pursuit of material wealth dominates people's lives. Global cultural trends like materialism, consumerism, hedonism, and individualism are harming moral values. In many subtle ways, people are drawn into serious kinds of human depravity, leading them to indulge in repulsive and abhorrent behaviors.

The culture of accumulating wealth, seeking power, and pursuing fame is harming how we live as humans in the world. This culture influences our sense of meaning and purpose in life, self-fulfillment, and the pursuit of happiness. The wealthy and powerful in society set examples for the poor of what happiness feels like. It has driven ordinary people to chase material prosperity at any cost.

The global culture is heavily influenced by relentless sensory stimuli.

Every day, we succumb to excessive desires and passions, becoming victims of fantasies and illusions of happiness. Most people fail to recognize the self-deceptions, life illusions, and childish fantasies they hold onto. They lose the moral sense and motivation that belong to the higher self and holistic personality.

In modern society, it is often clear that people do not understand why they act the way they do and struggle to discover who they truly are or are not. People set life priorities and goals and lead lifestyles driven by the culture of utilitarian individualism and a hedonistic approach to life. Many, caught under the spell of egoism, greed, and pleasure, develop thinking, emotional, and behavioral patterns that have no qualms about engaging in wrongdoing, regardless of how serious the harm to themselves or others.

In modern society, the 'hedonistic calculus' is frequently applied in the quest for success, happiness, power, and fame. An emphasis on individualism and a hedonistic outlook tend to drive people toward increasingly risky and troubling behaviors. Relying on this calculus can reduce one's appreciation for the aesthetic value of human life. Additionally, the mature moral self becomes less connected to everyday thoughts and actions, undermining its sense of purpose.

In the postmodern world, internet culture heightens the challenges to an individual's moral self. The harmful influences of the online environment increase the complexity of modern society's focus on individualism and hedonism. The rapid expansion of communication technology has introduced disruptive ideas that cause societal chaos and weaken social cohesion and the global order. The constant influx of new apps negatively impacts people's moral identities in ways that are often unnoticed, unacknowledged, or simply denied.

In our world, we are more connected than ever before. This means that events in one part of the world can greatly affect other areas. The ability to communicate instantly has made it easier for people to compare themselves to others. We quickly fall prey to the negative influences of strangers and develop harmful moral reasoning and motivations. We act prematurely without moral clarity.

Internet culture has created a slippery slope for personal morals. Online activities introduce new risks and uncertainties in moral judgment. Each day brings new challenges for responsible thinking, feeling, and behaving. Internet culture threatens people's consistent sense of self and identity. Online influences are the biggest obstacle to people's working self-concept and sense of self in modern society.

While we have gained a lot from the interconnected world, it also subtly and often unnoticed erodes our daily moral sense, reasoning, motivation, and behavior. In our society, it's widely accepted that the internet causes more confusion about moral issues, often leading to risky choices, decisions, and actions. Furthermore, online oppression, exploitation, and assault have become a new epidemic, significantly worsening moral decline in society.

The postmodern world reveals that people are overwhelmed by toxic division. In today's society, mutual trust is likely at its lowest point ever. Sociological researchers tell us that social trust is at an all-time low. Human culture shows that we lack the cooperation needed to come together and create solutions that can improve human lives for everyone. Instead, people are obsessed with ideologies and traditionalism. Modern society's individuals are conditioned by strict moral rationality and worldviews; they lack the broad perspectives that come from moral awareness.

Arguably, we are going through a particularly divisive period in our history. It is a time characterized by contentious debates and polemics that have marred human history. In these debates, people strongly defend their positions and are less willing to consider opposing viewpoints. This attitude has led some to believe they can freely infringe upon the basic human rights of others. It has fostered division and hostility among different societal groups. The hate, hostility, and violence rooted in society stem from polarizing ideas. When individuals become rigid and uncompromising in their moral beliefs, they tend to resist keeping an open mind and developing mutual tolerance and understanding. In a constantly changing world, evolving one's moral self is essential to stay receptive to diverse opinions and ideas, fostering mutual tolerance and respect for differences.

In modern society, the harmful moral character of people is best reflected by the ideological chaos present. It causes significant pressures, always threatening social cohesion and stability. Primarily, the degenerate moral environment in society results from ideological chaos. We see unproductive and unempathetic dialogue across ideological boundaries. Ideas often trigger emotions and behaviors that are deeply rooted in the human psyche and influence relationship patterns within society.

People's rigid moral self views the world in black and white. This moral perspective arises from a distorted and corrupted understanding of moral purposes and motivations that shape daily thoughts and actions. When the moral self is inflexible and underdeveloped, we see the world as a battlefield. Human life becomes a struggle between good and evil. We are willing to kill or die to achieve our version of utopia. This kind of moral self can motivate not only extremists but anyone vulnerable to it.

Today, we are neglecting urgent moral and social issues that demand our attention. We encourage the socially binding moral self to conform to specific worldviews, values, and attitudes by adopting a "fixed mindset" and resisting the "growth mindset" of the individualizing moral self.

With the "fixed mindset" of a rigid moral self, we fail to see that people, not ideologies, are the sources of solutions if we want to find new and better ways to live productively in the postmodern world. In contrast, the "growth mindset' reflects a more advanced, mature moral self that guides ideas and beliefs shaping daily thinking patterns. People with the "growth mindset" work to bridge divides and empower everyone around them.

When people lean toward arrogant righteousness, finding common ground becomes nearly impossible. When we cannot perceive existential truth and reality in the moral realm, the weak and inflexible moral self dominates over moral rationality and truth. We are unable to recognize objective truth and can only conceive subjective truth that serves our convenience.

What is becoming clear in our world is the relentless trend toward silencing critical and alternative viewpoints. The heavy-handed approach to dealing with dissenting voices is more common today. Our world tends to subjugate and dominate others, often causing serious harm to opponents instead of seeking understanding. We live in a world where horrific crimes are committed against those who oppose others' viewpoints. Sadly, it is all too common for opponents, rivals, and enemies to disappear entirely. It is the modus operandi of those in power to silence the "prophetic voice" of moral consciousness-driven people and truth-seekers in our society.

This has become a widespread problem in modern society. We are increasingly exposed to the complete depravity of many influential and powerful people. The danger lies in how desensitized we have become to it. The cruel and malicious actions of the powerful are reflected in the ripple effects of growing brutality spreading throughout society. The harmful influence of unconscionable and malicious individuals today encourages a culture of hate, vengeance, and deadly retribution. How opponents are treated in our society mirrors the terrible, vicious, and almost demonic moral state of our times.

Furthermore, we are used to people, both privately and publicly, constantly denying, avoiding, and twisting objective truth. This creates a new world order where there are no limits to what can be done, no matter how malicious, to prevent the truth from being exposed. It happens all the time, and most people passively, if not indifferently, accept it. This shows that we more easily drift away from existential truth and lean toward illusions and delusions. These illusions and delusions about life support people's moral behaviors. The behaviors demonstrate that living a life of contradictions has become the new normal in modern society. It reflects the human reality of the "new" human phenomenon in the postmodern world. Today, people tend to be frighteningly enigmatic and approach one another cautiously.

It is a well-known fact that a person's psycho-social environment affects their human consciousness. In modern society, people are influenced by the sensually driven aspects of their cultural surroundings. Sensuality now dominates human consciousness and has become its default state. Life experience shows that sensual cultural influences largely shape the level of human consciousness in everyday individuals. Cultural values and attitudes often do not guide people's attention toward self-sabotaging patterns of feeling, thinking, and behaving. Constant exposure to a sensual lifestyle gradually leads to self-destruction; yet, people often find themselves stuck in this difficult-to-change sensual mindset.

Imperceptibly, modern sensual culture erodes moral awareness, which could foster the development of the moral self. Each day, we try to hide the flaws of our harmful moral self and neglect personal growth. We live with a false sense of identity. Without self-evolution, we struggle to reflect a mature moral self of a wholesome, higher-quality person. We lack a complete understanding of self. Without a developed moral self, we fall short of becoming a better version of ourselves. We are unaware of who we truly are and who we can become.

The constant flow of harmful cultural influences continually challenges the integrity and consistency of individual identity and self-structure. Cultural factors in the postmodern era weaken the mature moral self and psychosocial growth required to resolve moral conflicts and issues. Consequently, many people we encounter daily lack moral clarity and experience profound inner turmoil.

Contemporary Human Self-Identity

An honest evaluation of people's behaviors in modern society indicates that the dubious, duplicitous, and dishonorable often reveal people's true selves from all walks of life. The actions of the cunning, unscrupulous, elitist, and hypocritical contribute to shaping the current perception of identity. We endorse attitudes and values that undermine everything good and noble. We go through life with only a false sense of self.

The modern idea of self is heavily influenced by current dreams and ambitions, which motivate people's pursuits of success, happiness, and self-fulfillment. We live in a world that, despite changing faster than ever, also makes moral clarity and purpose in our decisions more complex. Goals related to self-fulfillment considerably shape how people view themselves. Their choices, preferences, and decisions often focus on self-interest. The 'what-is-in-it-for-me' attitude drives many individuals in today's society. Modern psychology sees the culture of consumerism, individualism, and hedonism as eroding people's sense of self.[19]

In modern society, people's dreams and ambitions sometimes seem like they're straight out of a fairy tale. Usually, folks are constantly caught up in illusions of success and happiness. The feeling of delusional self-identity can harm the true self and lead people toward self-important pursuits. Dreams and ambitions often cause many wrongful actions in daily life. The moral logic of traditional morality usually doesn't support the growth of a higher self. Denying what is true and false about our authentic selves reveals a flawed, weak, or inflexible moral sense.

The most common issue of modern times is self-centeredness and its damaging effects on society. Self-centeredness is seen everywhere in our world.

---

[19] Kasser, T. The High Price of Materialism. MIT Press, Cambridge; 2002

It is universally experienced in all human situations today. Unlike the survival instinct of self-preservation, self-centeredness shows that people are overly self-absorbed. When someone is self-centered, they habitually prioritize themselves over others or anything else. Self-centeredness is a primary trait of people's thinking and behavior in society, reflecting the modern idea of selfhood.

In modern society, people live in self-imposed confinement and are caught in chaotic freedom, obsessively fantasizing and deceiving themselves every day. They find it impossible to break free from their self-centered interests, dreams, and goals rooted in illusions and fantasies. Although life's illusions and the delusional self lead to shame, despair, and tragedy, they resist facing their true selves and the purpose of human existence. The behavioral signs of people today show self-doubt, self-destruction, and self-sabotage.

The sense of self-centeredness in modern society ironically exposes that people are deeply ungrounded, unsettled, and self-alienated. Although self-centered individuals intentionally avoid shame, guilt, and disapproval in daily life, they constantly struggle with the pressure of fragmented personhood and trying to maintain their sense of self. Self-centeredness hinders the development of personhood and the growth of a complete self. The true self remains hidden in the shadows of daily self-incoherence and self-inconsistency. A misguided sense of self drives the ideas people form about what meaningful human existence is. They cannot find the sense of otherness within themselves to live from a higher level of personhood.

Utilitarian individualism—the strong tendency to see human life as a way to maximize self-interest at others' expense—is the most extreme form of self-centeredness in our society. It fosters an egotistical sense of identity based on harmful self-determination. Utilitarian individualism is the biggest obstacle to being other-focused in modern life. For many people today, it is challenging, if not impossible, to care about or show concern for others' well-being.

Utilitarian individualism significantly lessens respect and honor for what is human in others. It promotes lower standards for one's moral sense of personhood, negatively impacting self-perception in modern society. While utilitarian individualism may satisfy immediate needs, repeated reliance on it gradually leads to self-destruction, which manifests as a distorted sense of self.

The most serious consequence of utilitarian individualism is its adverse effect on a person's sense of self. It hinders the development of a better version of oneself. The harmful mindset promoted by utilitarian individualism largely shapes the "new" human identity in how modern people see themselves, which can become problematic for both individuals and society. The "new" human phenomenon in postmodern times often shows that people think and act without the purposefulness of a moral self. This distorted view of human identity shifts the focus away from pursuing higher ideals, purposes, and goals in life. Such a self-perception makes people less likely to build meaningful relationships based on interdependence and human solidarity.

When the behavioral tendencies of utilitarian individualism reflect one's moral abilities, it indicates a lack of moral clarity and reduced capacity for self-regulation. Harmful desires and uncontrolled impulses dominate the sense of self. We then become trapped in disorganized thinking, feelings, and behavioral patterns. This leads to self-conflicts, self-doubt, and self-inconsistencies, which have become more common experiences in people's sense of self. It is connected to the "new" human phenomenon in people's personality styles and how they function in daily life. The negative sense of selfhood arises from a moral self that cannot develop higher-order personhood.

Some mental health experts interpret the "new" human phenomenon using the DSM-V criteria for personality disorders. They observe thinking, feeling, and behavioral traits in people's sense of self that match the diagnostic symptoms of disorders such as borderline, dissociative, sociopathic, and narcissistic personality disorders. The increase of personality disorders in modern society is deeply troubling and threatening. It remains unaddressed in many individuals we live with and interact with daily—at home, at work, and almost everywhere else. When people dismiss the purposefulness of higher-level personhood, they tend to fall into thinking, feeling, and behavioral patterns that contribute to personality disorders.

Personality disorders often reflect a chaotic and problematic sense of self. The disturbed, distorted, and perverted self-perception results from the irrationality of the moral self, negatively impacting an individual's psycho-emotional and psychosocial well-being more than chemical imbalances, as many mental health experts suggest. Neuroscience shows that thoughts and emotions influence brain mechanisms and chemistry.[20] The widespread presence of personality disorders today is a significant obstacle to achieving goals that improve human life and prevent adverse consequences.

The self-assertions of people in modern society show that individuals often feel entirely free to choose how to live without worrying about the effects on others. People are comfortable and secure in their humanity, even when their callous actions indicate a total disregard for others. We have developed a moral outlook that mainly sees other people as just a means to an end. We lack the moral capacity for empathy, care, and altruism. We are compromised in the essential need we all have for one another for personal well-being and happiness. In today's view of selfhood, the human being has started to resemble a mechanical lever that pushes others to follow egocentric self-determination.

Generally, we often assume in daily life that a person's self-determination equals a self-centered attitude, beliefs, and actions, even when the common good requires their attention. Self-determination often reflects an egocentric mindset that is unconcerned with how its actions impact others. The illusion of selfhood increasingly prevents people from understanding concepts like "common suffering," "common humanity," and "common destiny."

---

[20] Oken-Singer, H. et.al. The Neurobiology of Emotion-Cognition Interactions. Front Hum. Neurosci. (Vol.9); 2015

In today's view of selfhood, we struggle to recognize what is genuinely human in one another. We overlook the importance of connecting with like-minded souls. We have weakened our ability to develop our humanity through interdependence and solidarity fully. The burden of people's self-centered tendencies hinders the pursuit of a life rooted in principles, ideals, virtues, and empathy. Instead of building bridges that unite us, we construct walls that divide. The tendency to resist being part of the web of life leads to feelings of meaninglessness, deep loneliness, and insignificance in society. The severe psychological and emotional issues of self-alienation and social isolation in modern society reveal that feelings of unworthiness toward others burden people's sense of self.

The moral self significantly influences a person's sense of self. In today's society, people's understanding of identity often weakens higher-level personhood. An inflexible, fragile, or undeveloped moral self hinders advanced thinking and actions that define who we are. Without the insight and judgment of a mature moral self, it's hard to see that most of the time, we're caught up in illusions about our identity and purpose. We believe falsehoods about why we exist and what makes the "good life." For many, it's hard to imagine a different sense of self because of the powerful societal and cultural illusions and false beliefs that cause them to live without proper moral direction.

In the postmodern world, we often seem indifferent to higher ideals and purposes. We overlook the benefits that stem from a mature moral self to inspire and guide us. Contemporary people's sense of self shows a limited ability for rational self-awareness, self-understanding, self-regulation, and self-determination. Self-discipline is a rare and notable virtue that only a few seem to possess today. The harmful and corrupt moral self in contemporary people's sense of self persistently influences their personality styles, integrity, and character. The everyday thoughts and behaviors people have suggest they lack the wisdom of higher-order personhood needed to develop a sense of holistic selfhood.

In short, we are constantly in denial of objective truth. We poorly evaluate existential realities, struggle to understand existential perspectives, avoid confronting existential struggles, and fail to see how we shape the future of human existence. Due to this inability to face the objective truth, more and more people in modern society reveal the complex new human reality.

The world we live in seriously undermines what is most needed in postmodern times—namely, harmony, human solidarity, and interdependence. Relativism establishes the moral order in our society, making one's sense of selfhood unexamined and unchallenged. Without a mature moral self, people follow distorted moral thinking and perspectives that favor an egocentric sense of self. Every day, personal preferences and life priorities demonstrate that others do not matter in the pursuit of self-fulfillment, which significantly hinders the development of an altruistic selfhood.

Without a sense of self rooted in a mature moral identity, we allow the postmodern world to turn us into victims of our own wild imaginations and troubled minds. Few realize that when they are confined within the realms of fiction and fantasy, they become trapped by endless self-contradictions and live lives full of inconsistency. This reveals how contemporary people's sense of self hangs by a fragile thread. This might explain why negative feedback and interactions often cause people to lose their sense of self easily.

In the postmodern world, it is a significant challenge for people to develop a complete sense of self. The rigid and unchanging moral self leads to self-destruction without us realizing it. Our self-perceptions are based on a false sense of identity, built on fragmented personhood. These perceptions distort what it means to be human and what is truly normal in human life—namely, that bridging the gap between the pseudo-self and the real self is an ongoing journey. Becoming a better version of oneself is always a work in progress.

When we do not actively commit to self-evolution as a lifelong journey, we often lack a realistic and objective view of personhood and a clear sense of self. Without self-awareness and self-understanding, people's sense of self can become distorted, if not delusional. This occurs when we are not intentional about developing the moral self to become a better version of ourselves in the world. Consequently, individuals live based on a static self-concept and self-identity that weaken society's moral fabric and overall well-being.

In modern society, we navigate life with a distorted sense of self. We form feelings of self-worth based on self-deceptions and biased self-perceptions. People's self-esteem often overinflates who they truly are. We usually only understand others through shallow and superficial interactions. Daily, incidents where an "ego bubble" bursts reveal people's falsehoods and hypocrisies, casting doubt on the value of their distorted self-image. This confusion about our true selves demonstrates how our delusional self-perceptions can harm both others and the world.

The postmodern world often feels disorienting—like not knowing what to do with one's life. Daily experiences reveal that many people are struggling, pretending to be someone they are not. Many exert excessive effort to hide their true selves. Modern society as a whole struggles with the neurosis of complex personhood, which results in an arrogant and hostile sense of self. Amid our own personality issues and disorders, we must cope with this syndrome in others.

The effects of modern people's distorted sense of self are numerous and sometimes complicated to understand. Personally, it leads to feelings of confusion and delusion in life. Society, however, sees this twisted self-perception reflected in social unrest, racism, bigotry, human trafficking, sexual violence, and widespread illegal drug addiction. Globally, conflicts, brutal wars, ethnic cleansing, genocides, crimes against humanity, and other threats to human survival reveal the worst aspects of this distorted self-identity, influencing the course of human history.

Contemporary individuals often struggle to see the hidden moral conflicts they face because their sense of self-identity blocks their view. Almost everyone shows indifference or reluctance to face personal issues related to an abnormal, corrupted, or evil moral self. The widespread feeling of meaninglessness today is fueled by internal moral battles within a person's identity. The rigid yet fragile moral self significantly impacts daily thoughts, feelings, and actions. This rigidity suggests that many are reluctant to cultivate a more mature moral identity. Without continuous self-improvement to grow as a person, we prevent the full development of a morally advanced self—something that the postmodern world requires.

On a more optimistic note, evolutionary theorists suggest that we are entering the next phase of natural evolution. They believe it involves a transformation of human consciousness. Some theorists propose that the phenomenon of the "new" human reality we experience today may indicate that humanity is in the process of rebirth.

Evolutionary theorists argue that current shifts in the human psyche indicate ongoing natural evolutionary processes. They believe that the preordained emergence of a new human consciousness, part of this natural evolution, presents unique challenges to the moral self. This forms the foundation for the struggle with higher-order personhood and the development of holistic self-awareness. They suggest that in postmodern times, humanity is entering a new realm of consciousness. They view the "new" human phenomenon as shedding a fresh layer of a broader, higher level of consciousness. Although the timeline of natural evolution is fixed, they assert that soon, human consciousness will likely unify people more than ever before.

Contemporary Health Issues

Personal health and welfare, along with society's well-being, are not the main pillars of human quality of life today. We are failing to work effectively toward a healthier humanity and a safer world.

Generally, daily healthcare issues get the least attention worldwide. The importance of holistic health isn't part of the criteria for the "good life." We do not think of the "good life" in terms of good health, healthy relationships, and living in a healthy world. We often overlook healthier lifestyles and healthcare habits as key factors that positively influence health.

For many people, pursuing the "good life" means ignoring the harmful and destructive effects of the moral self on health. Every day, people's moral attitudes, values, and actions build up moral pain and suffering that subtly affect physical, mental, and social well-being. We are often unaware of how moral pain and suffering negatively influence health. Usually, we underestimate the role of the moral self in health.

However, modern health sciences' multidimensional concept of health highlights the moral aspect of personhood and the moral self.[21] Health professionals recognize that the moral self is essential for behaviors that prevent disease and enhance well-being. Yet, people often ignore the moral self as the fundamental cause of everyday health issues, whether physical, mental, or social.

In everyday life, people often overlook the concepts of moral health and moral disease. We tend not to recognize moral health and moral disease as part of health-related phenomena that affect life. However, health sciences show that moral health is a vital aspect of overall well-being. Health experts, researchers, and scientists emphasize that the moral aspect of humans plays a key role in health and illness.

It is clear that modern health systems neither prioritize moral health nor consider illness as a significant health concern, nor do they see it as very important in healthcare and treatment. Many health providers fail to recognize moral health or disease as being critically important in the process of building

---

[21] Joye Y., Bolderdijk J. W. An exploratory study into the effects of extraordinary nature on emotions, mood, and prosociality. Frontiers in Psychology (Vol. 5); 2015.

and maintaining good health. Society's indifference to moral health or disease shows that we are not only neglecting to address the root causes of personal health challenges—whether physical, mental, or social—but also the overall health and well-being of society.

No matter how much someone tries to hide their depraved or harmful moral self or deny the presence of moral issues within themselves, it eventually comes to light. Health sciences highlight that hidden internal factors influence people's health. Modern medical and health research provides evidence that behaviors driven by the moral self are at least partly responsible for many diseases, including physical, mental, and social conditions.[22]

Ordinary people often fail to recognize the early signs of deep moral pain and suffering as a warning of potential health decline. Furthermore, as a society, we are poor at noticing that our collective moral suffering is the most urgent warning that we are heading toward a bleak future for humanity.

Moral disease affects every part of human life. The moral pain and suffering experienced today are deep and difficult for society to manage. This widespread moral distress should be seen as a major public health crisis. In our era, moral disease has become a global emergency on an unmatched scale.

What is becoming clear in modern society is that more people are at the mercy of an unfamiliar "psychic underworld." The evidence of this appears in people's erratic and toxic desires, impulses, behaviors, and relationship patterns. We have become numb to the negativity of our daily thoughts, actions, and interactions. We are insensitive to our own feelings and those of others. We ignore the negative effects that our complex "psychic underworld" has on our relationships, health, well-being, and happiness, as well as on others.

Life evidence shows that people struggle daily to survive in a world that

---

[22] Galea S. Well: <u>What We Need to Talk About When We Talk About Health</u>. Oxford University Press; 2019.

feels unfulfilling. They feel trapped in insignificance and irrelevance, believing they are inconsequential to the world. Most of us live in a world that oppresses our human psyche. In postmodern times, people are overwhelmed by the pressure to be someone; not being somebody is psychologically threatening to many. To achieve "success" in the world has come to mean becoming a famous star and celebrity. The demands on mortal humans are overwhelming and distressing to the human psyche. Many, heavily burdened by the expectations of family, friends, and society, feel an insurmountable sense of despair. The effects on physical, mental, spiritual, and moral health are often overlooked. It leads many to walk through the doors of death from drug addiction, overdose, and suicide.

Additionally, the overwhelming despair caused by constant misery in human life generally is leading people to act in ways that threaten harm to themselves and others. Despite society's moral values, the moral self that people hold has no hesitation about engaging in dangerous behaviors. The shocking statistics of suicide-homicides today highlight how becoming insignificant to others can seriously affect mental health. This trend is affecting people everywhere and reflects a decline in moral wellness.

Today, we show an attitude that neglects moral health. Our society's disregard for moral well-being is similar to how we treat physical and mental health. We turn our bodies into toxin dumps and our minds into garbage dumps, then seek treatment for the consequences. Likewise, we fail to develop a mature moral self or enhance moral health, and are then forced to seek help in rehabilitation centers, through court orders, prison, or suffer from the crippling effects of moral decay.

Furthermore, the daily work we do for moral healthcare is replaced by psychotherapy. What was once considered sinful is now called psychopathology or classified as a mental health disorder. Psychopathology is closely linked to problematic behaviors caused by moral suffering. The corrupted or malicious moral self underpins our self-destructive and harmful actions. Often, mental disorders essentially reflect the abnormal state of a person's moral self. While not all mental illnesses are signs of moral poor health or the result of a malignant moral self, even minor moral lapses can indicate psycho-emotional health issues.

Mental illness resembles moral disease in many ways. Experts assert that improving moral health aligns with enhancing mental health. However, they do not view therapy-based rehabilitation as an alternative to restoring one's moral self. Modern science shows that it requires a mature moral self to accept responsibility for daily moral choices, decisions, and behaviors that contribute to disease in physical, mental, and social health, as well as moral disease.

Although society holds the sick responsible for cooperating with treatment, as Talcott Parsons identified, the "sick role" exempts the sick from responsibility for their condition.[23] Calling out destructive behavioral patterns is difficult in a world where "ego-worship" functions more like a religion. Today, self-righteousness and the tendency to blame make it hard to recognize or accept one's behavioral disorders. The significant advancements in healthcare, through the development of personalized medicine, genomics, and precision medicine, will not truly transform how we approach healthcare without focusing on the moral self of personhood.

We fail to realize that the healthcare imperative to "save a life" must go beyond just saving the physical person (biological organism). To "save a life" must also include considering the moral, spiritual, and social aspects as essential parts of the person's life. Modern science helps us see that the core human realities of morality and spirituality are most relevant to physical, mental, and social health.

Typically, we pursue values, priorities, and behaviors in daily life guided

---

[23] Parsons, T. Social Structure and Personality. The Free Press; 1965

by the moral self framework of traditional morality. The harmful effects of moral decline at personal, societal, and global levels, along with the deteriorated moral environment in the postmodern world, suggest that traditional morality is not very effective in healthcare today. People's rigid moral self is proving inadequate in guiding them toward what promotes health and prevents disease. When we neglect self-improvement or undermine the need to develop a mature moral self, we face moral conflicts and dilemmas and live with unresolved moral problems and challenges, which are directly or indirectly connected to healthcare issues.

Holistic health, a healthier humanity, and a better world order require a moral self rooted in personhood, guided by moral consciousness. When people's moral self promotes health and discourages disease, it goes beyond usual concerns with conventional moral rules and duties. A mature moral self is always needed to cultivate values, attitudes, and behaviors that support health promotion and disease prevention in postmodern times, and importantly, to enhance the quality of human life for everyone.

Contemporary Value of Humans

Postmodernity has caused moral conflicts and dilemmas, leading people to struggle with what it means to be truly human. It is the perceptual uncertainties in the moral framework of human life that guide how people understand what it means to be human in our world.

In modern society, it's clear that people's daily attitudes, values, and behaviors reveal less about what it truly means to be human. We struggle to see the common humanity in each other. There's a vague, complex, and corrupt sense of being human in others. Every day, we navigate life by interacting with people who lack the qualities that define us as humans. They are disoriented, shady, unhinged, and threatening.

What is becoming clear about people in modern society is that few possess self-knowledge and self-understanding, and even fewer are self-directed in life. This shows in everyday life as people tending to be unpredictable, reckless, and impulsive. The materialistic, consumer-driven, and hedonistic orientations in life are confusing people about what it means to be human. The acquisitive attitude overshadows the self-transformative attitude that one relies on to be genuinely human.

Today, people face overwhelming pressures to succeed, gain power, achieve social status, and seek validation from others. The obsession with material goals and egoism blocks the potential to become the best version of oneself. Conventional morality's moral framework does not stop wrongdoing. We often have no hesitation in ignoring moral guidelines, legal laws, public policies, social rules, or moral ideals and principles. As a result, we frequently engage in behaviors that damage self-respect and human dignity.

In the postmodern world, the material aspects of human nature influence how people understand what it means to be human today. Without the spiritual part of human nature, we are becoming emotionless, senseless, and lacking a soul. This is demonstrated by the unrestrained human acting like an automaton.

The postmodern world has altered our understanding of what it means to be human. The automaton often characterizes our humanity as "feeling-less," "soul-less," and "sense-less." This reflects the everyday reality of human existence—both within ourselves and in our interactions with others. It exposes the negative aspects of the "new" human phenomenon that are common in modern society.

The human existential reality is rooted in dissociation from objective truth and the true nature of human existence by dismissing the idea of a metaphysical human nature. Today, we live without awareness of this metaphysical human nature, often misunderstanding what it means to be human. In postmodern times, illusions, delusions, and fantasies about life mainly shape people's human reality.

The metaphysical represents the core of human nature. The ontological reality provides the context in which human essence is developed and enriched. It reflects the human potential to go beyond the limits set on the human mind. The ontological reality not only reveals the entire human experience but also offers the moral foundation for human existence. Furthermore, the ontological reality greatly influences deontological obligations.

Without an ontological foundation, people ignore all moral standards that define what it means to be human and support human life. Without the resource of the metaphysical, a person's sense of self and personhood poorly reflects humanity's moral nature. This explains a human reality where people's moral identity is often confused and disoriented.

In a rapidly changing world, people do not live practically or responsibly. This is because they avoid confronting the shortcomings of the socially imposed moral self. This moral self confuses, constricts, and disorients people about what it means to be human in a fast-changing world. Daily life shows that people do whatever they want, even when it causes serious and irreparable harm to themselves and others. They feel a stronger sense of being free to act without consequences.

In modern society, the 'care-a-damn' attitude equates to people's sense of freedom. The corrupt and malicious moral self dominates the sense of selfhood and promotes harmful behaviors and evil deeds. Only a few understand that true freedom in human life always comes with the burden of duty and responsibility to oneself and others. These rare individuals reflect human potential and the qualities of higher-order personhood. They show the world how we should be human if we want to renew the moral environment in society.

Without a developed moral self, we neglect our moral obligations and responsibilities toward each other. We handle everyday moral dilemmas, conflicts, and urgent questions about what it means to be human in ineffective ways, which highlights the adverse effects of postmodernity. This demonstrates that people today lack the moral capacity to guide us toward a better way of being human. What makes humans uniquely different from animals—the moral nature of humans—is obscured by degraded personhood and distorted selfhood.

Most people endorse a static, undeveloped moral self that fails to promote the behaviors in the moral sphere that truly define what it means to be human. They can only envision the moral self associated with conventional morality, rather than the potential one that can emerge from moral consciousness.

The new challenges and problems of being human in our world require us to continually adapt our moral perspective to operate with atypical moral responsibility and obligation. It emphasizes moral awareness rather than normative morality. More than just lacking moral standards, people exhibit a diminished capacity for 'self-transcendence' that defines what it means to be human. This leads us to absurd and preposterous dreams and cravings, which negatively influence human behavior.

The moral foundation for building a healthier human life in the postmodern world requires a commitment to the principles of interdependence and human solidarity. Meaningful coexistence relies on human sensitivities focused on the welfare of others. Today, our world needs everyone to promote human solidarity in all situations, even when it might threaten oneself. Yes, shaping a humane and fair world order is always a complex task, but it is possible. For example, during tragic or devastating events and stories, people willingly empathize and collaborate to ease human suffering. This response in our times reflects a moral awareness that highlights human suffering and tragedy. Genuine human compassion is awakened!

It is the moral rationality of moral consciousness, not normative morality, that elevates people beyond mere existence. Conceptualizing the moral self, which aims for the common good, interdependence, human solidarity, and meaningful coexistence, is neither empty rhetoric nor a self-defeating attitude in life. Destroying the well-being of any other human is truly self-defeating. Today, we are living in a way that undermines each other's welfare, which is ultimately self-defeating.

Every day, often in ways we don't notice, we stubbornly think and act based only on our own preferences and freedoms, sometimes at the expense of others' well-being and even lives. In our society, chasing selfish, egotistical gains at any cost often leads to the destruction of the common good and human solidarity. Yet, we neither recognize nor admit that this is happening all the time.

To share a common humanity, we all have a responsibility not to deny others the opportunities they deserve in life. Primarily, we must recognize that basic human respect, honor, and freedom are rights every person possesses that can never be violated. We should agree that everyone not only has the fundamental right to life but also deserves a "good life," which includes material, psychological, and spiritual needs.

Life evidence shows us that we often neglect to commit to or prioritize equality in human life. Our moral ideals, principles, and laws affirm the undeniable truth that all are equal and entitled to fundamental human rights. However, people who vigorously defend moral ideals and principles also tend to avoid the moral responsibilities we have to one another in daily life. We deny and deprive our fellow humans of opportunities for a better quality of life each time we ignore injustices and inequalities. We violate basic human dignity and respect when we lose our sense of shared humanity by refusing to show compassion, tolerance, and mutuality. The common understanding that everyone shares a common destiny has made us indifferent to collective suffering. The way we live in the postmodern world suggests that we are apathetic and unconcerned with a global effort to enable all humans to enjoy life, liberty, and the pursuit of happiness.

The devastating consequence of modernity lies in how we understand what it means to be human. It is most evident in the dangerous worldviews people adopt by cherry-picking, decontextualizing, and ignoring the objective truth and the fundamental reality of human existence. This leads to treating one another as "objects" rather than as "subjects" with free will, rights, and self-determination. Those who embrace a weak, rigid, deviant, and destructive moral self have the most harmful impact on how they tend to be human in postmodern times.

The worldviews that people hold onto undermine the existential perspectives needed for interdependence, human solidarity, and meaningful coexistence. They weaken our ability to develop empathetic friendliness and virtuous behaviors. We do not aim to confront and solve everyday human challenges in society by reaching higher levels of personhood through cultivating our full moral capacities. The psychosocial maturity necessary to be truly human in the postmodern world requires everyone to commit to ongoing self-evolution as a lifelong process.

Many people in our world seem unaware that reaching full human potential depends on developing higher levels of personhood. This mainly involves cultivating a mature moral self and psychosocial maturity. Without a mature moral self to face modern moral conflicts and issues, we lack basic moral understanding and the responsibility to cherish the gift of life we have and to give to others. The most significant human achievement is recognizing that the actual value of one's life lies in being a gift to others through a commitment to their well-being.

The widespread problems of corruption, drug addiction, heinous crimes, and brutal killings in society constantly remind us that people often fall short of higher ideals and goals in life. The monstrous and evil tendencies of despots, authoritarian regimes, gang leaders, drug cartels, terrorist organizations, and similar groups warn us daily that the moral authority within oneself can lead to destructive consequences. The evil acts in our world send a loud and clear message: self-improvement and developing a mature moral self are essential choices.

The widespread issues of depression, aggression, and addiction in today's society are the "unheard cry for life's meaning and purpose," referencing Viktor Frankl. The distorted understanding of what it means to be human underpins a deep sense of meaninglessness, leading to many mental health problems. The struggle to be human in our times is pushing society to the brink of insanity.

The psychological signs of life's meaninglessness in today's world are evident in the neglect of moral duty and responsibilities to oneself and others. The harmful and destructive behaviors seen in addiction, self-abuse, crime, suicide, and homicide are also, if not more, indicators of people's sense of meaninglessness.

All of life's struggles and efforts are ultimately meaningless without a higher purpose and meaning. People's daily thoughts, feelings, and actions cannot exist in an existential vacuum. They can only be understood within the moral framework of a person's moral self. Usually, this moral framework in modern society encourages excessive self-indulgence and weak self-control, and discourages human empathy and kindness.

The meaning and purpose in a person's life are the primary motivating forces behind all human successes and failures. Believing that one's life is meaningless can imply that it is without purpose or has no worth to the individual. When we promote a sense of humanity that diminishes higher-level personhood, we distort the meaning of life and undermine human value in our world.

Life's meaning and purpose are better understood through higher-order personhood. The tendency to devalue and underestimate the priceless worth of human life today underpins all ethical issues, the widespread moral decline, and the corrupted moral environment in the postmodern world. The mature moral self serves as the key tool and motivating force to pursue a better version of personhood and a richer way of being human. The higher quality of human life in a person reflects holistic selfhood as the essential focus in how we are to be human.

WHAT COMPLICATES OUR MORAL SELF

The moral self of personhood reveals how someone exists as a human being in the world. Whatever is good, right, just, virtuous, divine, or bad, wrong, unjust, diabolical, and demonic in a person reflects the overtones of the moral self of personhood. The moral self is typically shaped by a person's historical, social, and cultural contexts. Usually, one's moral self adapts to changing life circumstances. Experientially, people's moral reasoning, motivation, and behavior change – for better or worse – in response to issues in the moral domain.

The postmodern world has brought unique challenges to people's moral identities, shaping their sense of meaning, purpose, values, attitudes, and priorities in life. Postmodernity has formed a moral self that makes people more confusing, unpredictable, and even risky. Today, we meet individuals who do not pursue higher ideals and goals in their lives. The moral self they adopt does not define them as having a higher-level personhood or a developed selfhood. Postmodernity has created a human experience without a clear purpose for the moral self.

Today, there is little clarity about what defines the moral self or a universally accepted moral framework. There are no clear criteria for evaluating each other's moral identities. How people view the moral self is easily swayed by demagoguery. The harmful influences of modern culture lessen the importance of one's moral identity. For most, the moral self is not a primary concern in how we think, feel, and act. Few pay attention to issues of moral healthcare as much as they care for physical healthcare.

As a society, we are becoming used to ignoring the personal and collective harm caused by the moral self. We not only fail to recognize that the moral self we adopt and the moral standards we follow are rooted in a morally corrupt history, but also overlook the serious consequences for future generations caused by today's moral reasoning. Evidence from life shows that the moral self guiding current generations is creating an uncertain future for human life and the planet.

We live in a world filled with hate, hostility, and division. Every day, human solidarity and peaceful coexistence are challenged by conflicts arising from communal, racial, cultural, religious, and political differences. The current moral, political, and social climate sharply divides society into a highly polarized "them vs. us" mindset. About half of the people in every community and nation believe that the "other side" is immoral and dangerously evil.

In modern society, we encounter a range of conflicting moral viewpoints that can often be confusing. Every day, we struggle with understanding what the common good truly is or question whether it even exists. In public, people express dedication to the ideals of the common good, but in private, their actions frequently reveal a moral self that doesn't quite match those aspirations.

In modern society, we navigate a chaotic life and must handle the moral complexities of people. Every day, we experience and survive moments characterized by startling behaviors that fall short of human respect, dignity, and humane standards. The unpredictable behaviors of people indicate that there is no moral clarity and that moral uncertainties, more than mood disorders, drive these actions. People are often unaware of what they are doing or why they do it.

In modern society, problems caused by a deviant and malicious moral self spare no one from the devastating consequences of reprehensible, loathsome, or brutal behaviors. Such behaviors happen even in places and among people one least expects. The aggressive and scornful actions of society's upper tiers reflect an underdeveloped moral self of personhood.

In modern society, people are not who they believe they are, claim to be who they are, or appear to be who they really are. The true self is often hidden behind many masks suited to each situation. Today, it is common to hear stories about a spouse, a parent, a child, a neighbor, a friend, a trusted mentor, a member of a social group, a coworker, a famous person, or a public figure who has led a secret life that others did not know about.

In modern society, the true self is often still hidden. A person's transparency is tangled in masks and cover-ups. People's personhood and self-identity are mysterious, obscured by many screens. As a result, we often feel justified in being cautious around others—whether they are highly respected members of society or outcasts and disbarred individuals.

In modern society, few aspire to the higher level of personhood that reflects positive character traits like integrity, honor, wisdom, temperance, virtues, high-mindedness, and shared responsibility. We rarely meet individuals who are highly principled and honorable, with noble attitudes, human virtues, captivating integrity, and a mature moral and psychosocial character.

In modern society, people often resist change and self-improvement. Few seek self-evolution to become a better version of themselves and grow as individuals. Instead, we have become skilled at using deceptions and facades to hide the raw truth of who we are. Meanwhile, we constantly live in fear of being exposed for our true selves.

What's even worse is that sometimes, even when people are caught, they justify their actions and succeed in their wrongdoing. News media reveal evil-doers, whether famous or notorious, without shame, guilt, remorse, or self-control. They arrogantly display spiteful stubbornness despite the disastrous problems they cause for others and the world. These moments highlight people's self-righteousness, arrogance, and shameless defiance, vividly exposing the vicious moral self at work in society.

For many, especially among public figures and the renowned, being duplicitous, hypocritical, and leading a double life is a common way of living. Every day, people's duplicity and hypocritical behaviors reveal the emptiness of their moral selves. The double life of individuals is often suspected of hiding a closet full of skeletons. Clinically, the two-faced fraudster shows symptoms consistent with personality disorders.

In modern society, the moral self that people promote often disrupts their sense of identity. Self-incoherence and self-disintegration indicate that society undervalues the mature moral self. Many are driven to create and defend a self-image that attracts attention and respect from others, even when deep inside they feel threatened by who they are not and who they truly are.

This is a fact that is reflected daily by the disconnect between what people say and do, who they truly are, and how they want others to see them, along with how they live and want others to believe they live. The reluctance to face the "real me" directly highlights people's problematic human selfhood in modern society. The desperation to maintain a favorable social status and moral standing, despite their wrongdoings, suggests that people do not prioritize or genuinely care to understand their moral self, which guides their actions. This situation among people in modern society shows that we are trapped in the shallow aspects of human existence.

In modern society, the idea of a twisted and corrupted human selfhood is the least of people's concerns. Without the moral aspect of our personhood, the human soul ceases to exist as a self. The breakdown of people's personhood and distorted selfhood today reflects the struggle with the soul. The experience of people's fractured personhood and warped selfhood represents the chaotic human whose soul is in limbo.

The evidence of a corrupt heart and the twisted human core reveals the total depravity of the human being. Restoring one's soul involves the effort to reclaim one's rightful place in the natural world, as described in ancient writings as being the crown of creation. It is about restoring our human dignity within the animal kingdom.

In modern society, one might even suspect that few people care about the effort required to develop higher-order personhood. It is rare to encounter individuals who excel in life through righteous living and virtuous actions. We praise people as role models only for their skills, achievements, and artistic performances, not for maintaining consistent virtue and humaneness, which truly make them stand out in life. We judge a person's greatness by superficial aspects rather than by the transparency and authenticity of their character.

In modern society, many individuals gain fame in areas like business, sports, sciences, entertainment, or other fields; however, few are recognized for high integrity, virtuous character, psychosocial maturity, or human greatness. Forbes often does not feature people acknowledged for their humanity, higher-order personhood, or holistic selfhood. Does this imply that qualities such as humaneness, decency, integrity, character, virtues, high-mindedness, noble service, and empathetic humanity are less valued in our world?

There is an essential question for us to consider today: Are we indifferent to qualities of higher-order personhood, higher ideals, and higher life purposes, or do they no longer hold significance?

Some social critics argue that today, human life has become a playground for the rogue moral self. Every day offers a chance for the evil lurking beneath our constant tendency toward self-deception, denial of objective truth, and scheming behaviors. We stubbornly deceive ourselves and others about everything to mask the insecurities of fragile personhood and unstable self-identity.

Mental health experts argue that revealing one's moral self can threaten the psycho-emotional core of personhood, which may explain the bluntness of brazen defenses, denials, and disordered personality styles. They believe that without the mental capacity needed for self-evaluation and self-growth, people often justify being someone they are not. Evidence from real life shows that individuals who resist self-development tend to have a rigid, weak, or harmful moral self, but not a mature moral self or a sense of complete selfhood.

In our time, how people tend to be human shows that the moral aspect is fragile and delicate, and the moral self becomes disconnected from true selfhood. We are indifferent to the static, rigid, deviant, and malicious moral self that influences everyday moral sense, reasoning, and motivation for actions. This is the moral self that is always linked to the individual's working self-concept and self-identity as a person, and it is deeply involved in people's health, quality of life, and societal well-being.

A clear consequence of modern life is that more people accept a superficial human existence. We avoid authenticity and self-transparency. We do not feel motivated by the purposefulness of the moral self. We lack the drive to develop higher-order personhood to improve humaneness, integrity, and character. We settle for less in cultivating the mature moral self and psychosocial maturity of personhood. All of this shows indifference to one's human soul.

Modernity has shaped a new human reality, one that is less influenced by the spiritual and metaphysical and more by the physical, sensual, and material. The material aspect of human nature dominates human life. Evidence from life shows that for most people, reaching higher-order personhood is not within the scope of being human.

Cultural anthropologists, sociological experts, and health researchers observe that in postmodern times, global culture is effectively increasing abnormal behaviors in how we are human.[24] There are unique irregularities and abnormalities in what defines being human in postmodern civilization. Internet culture, utilitarian individualism, and hedonic life orientation negatively impact people's humanity in modern society.

In these postmodern times, widespread moral decay significantly disrupts human life. In modern society, the decline of moral integrity is most evident in people's self-deceptions, self-centeredness, and self-importance. Medically, it appears as extreme neurosis and psychosis in human nature today. It exposes a deviant, corrupt, and harmful moral self that negatively impacts how we exist as human beings.

A healthier humanity and a better world will remain just a distant dream as long as moral diseases worldwide do not go into remission. People's intense experience of overwhelming moral pain and suffering today is probably unknown to past generations. The widespread issues of addictions, suicides, homicides, and mental health problems like depression and anxiety in modern society show that moral disease is ongoing. People are trapped in psychosocial-emotional troubles, damaging society's health and well-being.

It's important to emphasize that higher-order thinking, noble living, and virtuous relationships are essential tools in human life. These tools of higher-order personhood are always necessary and cannot be lost. A person's higher-order personhood relies on a mature moral self, particularly for psychosocial maturity, to shape how we are meant to be human in the world.

People's higher-order personhood and mature moral self are vital for making the world better for everyone. However, what stands out most in our world is that few people are willing to self-evolve, develop morally, and grow in psychosocial maturity by learning from daily life experiences the "truth

---

[24] McInnis, H (Editor) Utilitarianism and its critics. MacMillian Publishing Company; 1990. Mousavi, Asl SM. et.al. Psychology of Ethics. Qom: Research Center and University; 2016.

phenomena," which offer lifelong lessons.

Everyone's personal history can teach us what is needed to find inner freedom, peace, and happiness. Usually, we know many things, but we understand little and only superficially about our own history. When we give in to harmful cultural influences, most people's histories become buried under intense psychological, emotional, and social complexities.

As humans, we are born to learn valuable wisdom through life experiences, but often fail to grow in wisdom. In the constant struggle for self-preservation, nearly everyone overlooks the importance of honoring the moral self of personhood. However, it is this moral self that can help us find truth and teach us that, through life experiences, there are many lessons to learn about how to develop higher-level personhood.

To better understand people's moral selves in modern society, we need to analyze (1) institutional moral rationality, (2) self-fulfillment goals, and (3) the public moral self.

Institutional Moral Rationality

Usually, we rely on the moral framework of traditional morality to guide us through life. It reflects society's institutional moral reasoning. Today, people's moral thinking often aligns with outdated moral rationality. In a very complex world, the moral perspectives we hold onto are proving ineffective and irrelevant for solving current problems, issues, and challenges in the moral realm.

Whether we realize it or not, we have inherited a legacy of rigidity and stubbornness in the moral reasoning that guides modern life. We adopt the Pharisaic, highly critical, guilt-ridden, and harm-focused thinking patterns from past generations. Moreover, moments in history like colonialism and slavery continue to influence the present. The calls for restorative justice from survivors and victims of past atrocities not only echo the moral irrationality of those times but also reveal similarities with our current era.

Today, we develop a moral self that allows us to justify our wrongful acts and avoid taking responsibility. The significance of moral human nature is often downplayed in modern society. People's behavior typically does not reflect the qualities of a mature moral self. Daily actions in society demonstrate less evidence of the psychosocial maturity that underpins higher-level personhood and a complete sense of self. We observe that individuals, regardless of their background or social status, are unpredictable and dishonorable. It appears that simply holding on to abstract ideals of traditional morality has left us fragile, capricious, and unchangeable.

There is no doubt about the influence of the moral self on a person's personality and sense of identity. Our daily actions clearly demonstrate that the moral self we adopt can either positively or negatively affect how we experience being human in the postmodern world. It is the main factor that shapes or distorts what it means to be human. What is obvious through people's working self-concept and self-identity is the absence of a mature moral self in understanding how to be human. A weak, rigid, or harmful moral self exposes the everyday struggles of people's distorted sense of self.

Modernity has gradually diminished a sense of self rooted in core human virtues and empathetic kindness. Each day, this decline is reflected in how people view themselves and how they treat others. We demonstrate less compassion and see one another as if we are interchangeable objects. Evidence of this is visible in the harshest cruelty inflicted on fellow humans in modern society. The fragile, inflexible, and often malevolent moral self—if not outright malicious—influences daily behavior, usually justified by institutional moral rationality.

It is often observed today that people's public personas do not reflect who they are in private settings or roles. The emphasis on the moral rationality of social institutions weakens, rigidifies, and underdevelops the moral self. Who one is or what position one holds in society does not ensure a mature moral self. Each day, we see individuals with a fragile moral core of personhood. This highlights that little importance is placed on the inherent moral capacity of human nature for developing personhood and selfhood. We tend to overlook the moral foundation that supports strength and consistency in personhood. People are often guided by moral rationality that can lead to feelings of instability in personhood and a distorted sense of self. This can result in problematic behaviors with serious consequences for society, to which many are indifferent or unaware.

Almost everywhere—at home, at work, or in public—we encounter people who are unstable and erratic. They display a sense of inconsistent identity, reflecting a distorted self-perception. Although many try to appear strong and composed, inwardly they are fragile and fragmented. Many are on the brink of collapsing into the abyss of deindividuation. In a world where a pill can fix everything, it is psychotropic medication, more than self-improvement or the strength of integrity and character, that keeps people resilient and strong internally. In modern society, people reveal that the human self is less a unified identity. Daily experiences of self-inconsistency and incoherence point to a widespread neglect of essential spiritual and moral human realities in our way of living.

There is concern about the experience of postmodernity and the way of life it has brought about. In the postmodern world, we generally go through life without aiming for higher development of personhood. We ignore moral health and think less about what it truly means to be genuinely human. The media often expose even moral authority figures who appear to be calm and composed in their daily lives, yet are driven by a harmful and terrible moral self.

In today's multicultural society, it's believed that each culture has its own equally valid morality. However, in modern society, all moral systems are heavily influenced by outdated ideals, norms, and rules. These moral rules, developed over many years, often make moral reasoning more complicated and can hinder the motivation for behaviors that the modern world requires.

For most people, traditional morality is seen as the only limit to developing the moral self. However, the moral reasoning behind traditional morality is becoming ineffective in today's rapidly changing world. It not only shapes their moral worldview—many of which are no longer relevant in postmodern times—but also creates opportunities for wrongdoing and evil. Conventional morality often confuses realistic moral reasoning when people face moral issues today. Due to the ambiguity in moral reasoning within this framework, people usually feel no guilt about committing evil acts, harmful behaviors, and inhumane treatment of others.

In many situations in life, the norms, principles, and ideals of conventional morality do not support the growth of healthy personhood, a better humanity, or an improved world. Institutional moral rationality subtly and indirectly encourages us to engage in self-deception and deny objective truth. Often, however, the moral self may be feigned to make people appear as what they are not; the consequences of the fake moral self cannot be hidden. In their daily thoughts, feelings, and actions, people fail to see the rough edges and cracks all around them. They tend to disconnect from who they truly are and what they genuinely stand for.

The mindset shaped by the moral rationality of social institutions lacks the critical thinking needed to confront the objective truth. Despite this, people claim moral independence by adhering to institutional moral rationality. They are content with rigid black-and-white moral reasoning that often conceals what is truly despicable and abhorrent in their actions and behaviors. Institutional moral rationality supports the goal of saving face and presenting a moral self that aligns with society's standards. It encourages people to create an ideal moral persona, mainly to gain others' approval, even if they are fundamentally corrupt. Today, the corrupt moral self in a person is not only hidden from others but also from themselves, obscured by a twisted sense of self.

Primarily, conventional morality aims to avoid criticism, getting caught, or condemnation. Every day, people focus on following moral standards to appear moral and decent. The primary objective of a person's moral self is to uphold the appearance of doing what is right to meet societal expectations for human decency, even when the questionable behaviors are unconvincing. The moral self mainly serves ego needs rather than striving for higher personal growth and improving life for everyone. Daily behaviors often do not reflect the intention or goal of promoting the common good and a better life for all.

In everyday life, when an individual's moral capacity is limited by the intense demands of traditional morality systems, it impacts the objectivity and rationality that support motivation and behavior. Often, we find ourselves unable to choose for or against the ideals, principles, values, attitudes, and behaviors outlined by morality. This demonstrates that institutional moral rationality is not only ineffective in moral matters but also obstructs the development of a mature moral self and psychosocial growth essential in postmodern times.

What is clear today is that the standards established by traditional, conventional, and normative morality systems for one's moral self hinder practical moral understanding and motivation toward common human goals. From a strictly logical point of view, without a higher purpose in life, the development of a mature moral self and personhood is suppressed. People generally demonstrate a mature moral self and psychosocial maturity—reflected through higher-order personhood—when they are intentional in their connection to the web of life. The ideals and purposes of higher-order personhood challenge the worldviews that lead us into black-and-white moral thinking.

In a constantly changing world, the rigid moral reasoning of social institutions shapes society's overall moral health. The bureaucratic logic of these institutions dominates society's moral framework and is deeply embedded in how people think about morality in their daily lives. Cultural critics and scholars recognize that society's stubborn insistence on the moral rationality of social institutions makes people's moral selves vulnerable to confusion.[25] There is no definitive moral truth—only conflicts and dilemmas in the moral realm. By fixating on traditional moral ideals and principles, we are prevented from perceiving the objective truth and reality, even when it is right in front of us.

The thinking and emotional patterns formed by institutional moral rationality confuse us, much like being lost in a confusing alleyway. When bureaucratic truth controls the moral framework, people encounter moral chaos, and urgent moral issues remain unresolved. The routine boredom with institutional moral rationality causes "moral fatigue" in people. They act based on their moral self, ignoring moral and legal laws, norms, and standards. This is shown by the widespread illegal, corrupt, antisocial, and vile behaviors in society, which harm everyone.

Bound by the moral rationality of social institutions, we lack the fully developed moral self and psychosocial maturity necessary to be completely human in the moral landscape of postmodern times. Often, in morally complex situations, the actions of the rigid, malicious, and underdeveloped moral self diminish what it means to be human. It is marked by the inconsistency of personhood and the instability of self-identity, undermining higher-order personhood. The true potential of one's moral capacities to become the human person one is can be poorly expressed when people's behaviors are erratic, deceitful, and outright harmful. This human condition results from the inherent moral nature being hindered, preventing us from reaching the objective truth. Our higher cognitive and emotional abilities are always at work, guiding us to

---

[25] Nowak, E. What is moral competence and why promote it? Ethics Progress (Vol. 7); 2016
Mercier, H. & Sperber, D. The Enigma of Reason. Harvard University Press; 2017

act with humanity.

Negatively, this fact is shown by the mistreatment of weak and vulnerable members of society, socio-economic disparities, racial and ethnic discrimination, and the disturbing statistics of brutal crimes, suicides, and homicides. The evil acts in our world, which seem endless, are hidden by the moral rationality of social institutions. The legal, political, and economic systems exploit and profit from the moral rationality of these institutions.

The main problem with institutional moral rationality is the moral suffering it causes without us realizing it as the root cause. Today, we must evaluate how social institutions serve as tools for shaping people's moral selves, considering human life quality and humanity's future. What is clear in modern society is that individuals who respond more effectively to moral problems and challenges do so by developing their innate moral abilities rather than relying solely on conventional morality.

When the moral rationality of conventional morality and social institutions dominates people's moral self, they become limited by the moral worldviews it creates. There is little evidence of attitudes, values, and priorities that foster empathetic friendliness and human solidarity. When firmly rooted in a prescribed morality, people diminish the natural potential—the higher cognitive and emotional capabilities—of human nature to develop a mature moral self and personhood. In today's world, it is essential to tap into the moral capacities inherent in human nature rather than relying solely on abstract ideals of conventional morality. The mature moral self, not the rigid one, mainly demonstrates what it means to be truly human in postmodern times.

Today, people are deeply immersed in illusions and delusions about life. Denying existential truth and reality creates more psychological and emotional challenges, struggles, and problems that we might not notice. Many in modern society live as if in a fairyland, far from true existential reality. Although fleeting, existential truth is incredibly valuable because we find it only in real-time life. It takes a mature moral self—one that is undeterred by societal moral rationality and truth—to grasp the present-moment existential truth.

People's mature moral self engages in life with higher cognitive and emotional abilities to understand the complexities of moral issues and reach the full depth of existential truth. The potential of our innate moral capacity exceeds the limitations imposed by bureaucratic reasoning about truth. Only by developing the higher cognitive and emotional abilities unique to human nature can we become skilled at uncovering the raw existential truth in each present moment, especially in the moral realm. This mature moral self within a person plays a crucial role in fostering harmony and peace within because we align with the objective truth.

The reliance on bureaucratic reasoning about truth hinders people from fully understanding existential reality. We forget that achieving self-maturity, higher-level personhood, and societal well-being depends on being open to rational, objective existential truth. To become morally relevant and effective in society, one only needs to respond to the present-moment existential truth, fact, and reality in the moral realm. The ability to address immediate moral issues honestly reveals what is truly deep and authentic in a person. That is what makes someone genuinely human in postmodern times.

Today, we navigate the perilous waters of evil in the world. Institutional moral rationality is often used to justify antisocial actions rather than fostering the development of a mature moral self that enables the psychosocial growth the changing world demands. People's moral self tends to prioritize face-saving tactics over self-improvement and human development. They hide behind institutional moral rationality, even when behaviors clearly harm the greater good. Locked in a rigid, static moral self, people's moral rationality cannot develop comprehensive perspectives when faced with moral dilemmas and conflicts.

We are either neglecting the monarchial rule of the moral self over our humanity or ignoring the consequences of behavioral anomalies in society. When people feel secure in institutional moral rationality, they become indifferent to everyday harmful and destructive psycho-emotional and behavioral patterns. Modern psychology views destructive thinking patterns, psycho-emotional upheavals, and erratic, reckless behaviors as signs of self-disintegration in an individual. Life evidence indicates that today, self-disintegration processes in individuals are more prominent than self-integration ones. The rigid, weak, and malignant moral self of personhood underpins the experience of people's sense of a distorted and delusional selfhood.

There is a clear divide between the moral self needed to heal the world and the one derived from conventional morality. Usually, few recognize the elements within themselves that hinder healing. Most people resist examining and understanding the moral self that guides their lives. We often overlook the importance of each other's moral selves. We tend to be confident about our own moral self. As a result, it's easier to look down on or dismiss others simply because they have a moral self with different reasoning from ours. Without a mature moral self, we have less connection to the shared humanity that unites us all.

When people focus on personal preferences, driven by a rigid, weak, or undeveloped moral self, they behave irrationally. As a result, we often see individuals lacking a sense of connection to shared humanity, as seen in previous generations. This is evident daily through societal behaviors fueled by hatred, hostility, and sociopathic tendencies. Many individuals in our world can be described as cold, indifferent, and hard-hearted. Numerous unimaginable life situations reveal behaviors that are even considered psychotic by medical and legal standards. When the greater good is overshadowed by moral irrationality, it undermines higher goals for human life and the future of humanity.

Institutional moral rationality limits people's ability to foresee the consequences of their actions, reducing the purposefulness of the moral self.

Today, this issue appears as moral chaos, conflicts, dilemmas, and confusion. Following institutional moral rationality often results in moral dilemmas, unresolved ethical questions, and moral pain and suffering for individuals, along with moral decline worldwide. This happens because we develop our sense of a moral self through life experiences, which many find leads to a feeling of life's meaninglessness. Few realize that their moral confusion, unresolved social problems, and human suffering in society affect future generations. With a reduced moral capacity to protect the well-being of future generations, we show a weak commitment to humanity's and the planet's future. Daily dreams, ambitions, hopes, and drives of ordinary people often go unnoticed, yet they have a significant influence on the future. This demonstrates how others usually disregard the human depravity of today's generation.

By focusing solely on the present, we are dismissing any hope for a definite future for upcoming generations. The effort to safeguard humanity's future, which remains a controversial topic in society, is based only on current standards of institutional moral reasoning. Public conversations about the future often reveal opinions, logic, and emotional reasoning that lack the nuanced understanding of the significant harm that will probably occur later. As a society, we lack a clear, intentional goal to ensure a better future for ourselves and future generations.

Modern priorities, ambitions, and goals for human life make it seem like our thoughts and actions have little impact on future generations. We demonstrate moral reasoning that only meets the basic needs of the vulnerable and a rigid moral self focused on protecting future generations. However, when people prioritize self-improvement and higher-level personhood, their thinking, perceptions, values, and attitudes all encompass broader global perspectives within the moral domain. Future generations expect this from each of us.

Through self-evolution, we unlock the inherent potential of human moral nature. Human growth and the development of personhood are essential for enhancing the moral abilities of a mature moral self and achieving psychosocial maturity. An individual's moral self must evolve and mature to develop better moral understanding and motivation if they are to respond effectively to the challenges of modern life. Primarily, the renewal of the moral self begins with people questioning the relevance of traditional moral standards, ideals, and norms, as well as the moral rationality of social institutions that influence everyday human life.

Self-Fulfillment Goals

The socio-cultural factors unique to the postmodern world have the most significant influence on today's generations. Global cultural phenomena like consumerism, hedonism, and individualism are forces that shape our daily attitudes, values, dreams, ideals, and motivations. The human culture of the postmodern era can be described by insatiable greed, hedonistic pursuits, illusions of happiness, and childish fantasies, which drive people's goals for self-fulfillment. These elements support the hypocrisy, deception, and illusions of people's self-identity.

The contextual framework of the world is crucial to how we find meaning, purpose, and goals in life. Today's global culture tends to pull people toward superficial and unnecessary things. In modern society, people's lifestyles, priorities, and goals often revolve around self-promotion and seeking validation through social power and status. No matter how much material wealth we accumulate, it never feels enough. The superficial aspects of life divert attention from core human realities, such as moral and spiritual dimensions, as people set goals for self-fulfillment.

Usually, one's sense of self is shaped by the dominant culture. The intricate relationship between human selfhood and social influences is reflected in people's values, priorities, and goals. These values, priorities, and goals make up the moral framework that guides daily feelings, thoughts, and actions. The existence of a corrupt and harmful moral self in society shows a moral framework that strongly rejects higher ideals, higher purposes, and the common good.

In today's world, people's moral framework in daily life is heavily influenced by the surrounding environment of a morally declining society. The moral self of an individual constantly interacts with the world, either positively or negatively. It isn't easy to focus on the moral self without also considering the conditions that support it. Conversely, we struggle to understand the world unless we are continuously developing a mature moral self. What stands out most in modern society is that the moral self of personhood is often the least of one's concerns.

Modernity has brought wealth, prosperity, and abundance to more people than ever before. Material success, accumulating wealth, and pursuing pleasures are key drivers of self-fulfillment. In contemporary society, wealth, fame, and power are viewed as symbols of the "good life," widely regarded as desirable. Self-fulfillment is often achieved when someone attains a higher social status linked to wealth, power, and fame, but not necessarily moral integrity, character, good health, meaningful relationships, or an enriching quality of human life.

A materialistic and greedy mindset leads people into a life full of fantasies, illusions, and delusions. In our world, we chase success, happiness, and self-fulfillment, which often turn out to be illusions and fleeting dreams. As is usually the case, we tend to realize this truth too late. It is rarely considered that when fantasies, illusions, and delusions guide a person's journey through life, the cost is paid in personal health, well-being, and relationships. Most importantly, it can also prevent an other-centered approach that could improve society's health and welfare.

The grand dreams and goals of self-fulfillment fuel self-centered thinking and behavior patterns. In the postmodern world, few realize that the pathological self-centeredness flourishing in society underpins people's social attitudes and moral character. They often exhibit a more malignant and corrupt moral self that influences life goals, ethical choices, and lifestyles. This frequently results in an abnormal sense of self and a delusional identity that contribute to chaos and disorder in life.

People's moral framework aligns with their goals for self-fulfillment. Moral reasoning, judgment, and motivation that impact self-fulfillment may depend on either the static or evolving moral self within a person's identity. In modern society, it is clear that the static, undeveloped moral self often leads to illusions of self-fulfillment. An individual's needs for self-fulfillment increase or decrease depending on how human they are in the world. The moral self, which influences people's priorities and goals, is essential to how they think and behave as humans.

In modern society, self-centeredness and utilitarian individualism shape people's pursuit of self-fulfillment, driven by a sense of entitlement and intense envy. Although hard to accept, it is clear that today, people are pathologically motivated by self-centeredness. This mindset has made it difficult for individuals to distinguish right from wrong and good from evil.

In today's society, self-centeredness and utilitarian individualism driven by the pursuit of self-fulfillment have become widespread issues. It is a serious moral illness caused by egotistical greed, desires, and entitlement that is spreading faster than ever. This problem is the leading cause of abnormal behaviors, crimes, violence, and numerous social issues. It mainly contributes to the decline of moral values in society.

In modern society, people are experiencing a chaotic "inner world" caused by harmful cultural influences. The complex interaction between culture and psycho-emotional processes becomes clear as individuals become more inconsistent, unstable, and unreliable. Sociocultural influences generate numerous moral uncertainties, negatively affecting a person's psycho-emotional health and leading to abnormal behaviors. This indicates that self-evolution and the mature moral self are not solely part of one's self-fulfillment.

Socio-cultural factors significantly influence and shape an individual's self-fulfillment needs and goals. Modern values, priorities, and aspirations define the framework of the moral self. It is clear in today's world that people encounter ethical and moral dilemmas that deeply impact daily life choices, decisions, behaviors, lifestyles, health, and more. We find it challenging to accept that self-fulfillment should always encompass good health, happiness, and an improved quality of life.

One's fundamental human needs for good health, personal well-being, and a holistic life are essential in the pursuit of self-fulfillment. Those dedicated to self-evolution believe that the potential of the mature moral self to achieve self-fulfillment goals is even greater than the "prosperity" of self-centered individuals. They demonstrate that self-evolution aligns with a higher level of self-fulfillment than what is driven by society's standards of the "good life." When the mature moral self pursues self-fulfillment goals, the goals based on society's standards of the "good life" become less appealing. Superficial and unnecessary things are seen as merely creating illusions of self-fulfillment.

People who evolve, grow, and change demonstrate that the goal of self-fulfillment always involves developing higher-level personhood, holistic health, and the well-being of others. They are tapping into the full potential of human nature in being human and living. They are not burdened by societal ideas and standards of the "good life." They find a more profound sense of contentment by being free from insatiable greed and constant egotism. They are not pressured by socio-cultural constraints that can distract them from self-reflection, self-integration, and self-growth. They correct the malign psychology of the delusional self, thereby improving health and happiness for everyone.

Often, on the surface, the moral self may seem to have little connection to self-fulfillment. However, this is not true! When everyday life matters are not viewed within the moral framework related to personal health, the quality of human life, and the welfare of society and humanity, we fail to recognize the importance of the mature moral self and do not distinguish it from the static, rigid, underdeveloped version.

When the static, undeveloped moral self becomes the moral agent in life, a person becomes vulnerable to self-delusions and illusions about life. We develop psycho-emotional patterns of the mind and psychosocial behavioral tendencies that cause harm rather than healing. This reflects the experience of the moral self in people's personhood, impacting the quality of human life and society's welfare today. Evidence from life suggests that the unscrupulous moral self acts as the moral agent influencing and controlling people's involvement in social, cultural, and political matters.

Health literature provides strong evidence that people's problematic behaviors directly harm society's health and well-being. Modern society struggles to handle issues causing chaos daily, including violence, crime, corruption, illegal drug use, and more. Problematic behaviors indicate that daily healthcare often overlooks the importance of moral self and moral health in achieving self-fulfillment.

Whether one recognizes it or not, most of us live without a clear purpose. People are motivated by the moral self that diminishes the intrinsic value of human life. Every day, we distort the meaning and purpose of our existence through self-centeredness. Our sense of life's meaning and purpose poorly reflects a tendency toward an other-centered life orientation. The principles of interdependence and human solidarity are not the main goals of our human existence. We hinder higher ideals and purposes with self-deceptions, illusions, and false beliefs.

When a person's sense of self is deeply rooted in traditional morality, their goals of self-fulfillment tend to focus on external things. These are usually linked only to fleeting whims, desires, and ambitions. The moral self protects a person's attitudes, values, and behaviors that they avoid confronting. We bypass moral conflicts and dilemmas by retreating into moral doctrines, traditions, and beliefs. We tend to avoid the more urgent moral issues at both personal and societal levels. We are least concerned with how we pursue human life's fulfillment, individually and collectively, which seriously endangers the planet and future generations.

No desire, ambition, or drive for fulfilling human life can be reasonable without acknowledging the existential truth. Facing this truth helps define what it means to be human in postmodern times. Recognizing the reality of our human existence places responsibility on us for the outcomes of our choices. Essentially, existential truth enables us to develop higher levels of personhood, a mature moral self, and psychosocial maturity that give life its meaning and purpose, shaping our goals for self-fulfillment.

Most often, we don't realize that the moral self rules like a monarch over who we are, how we act, and where we're headed in life. When guided by conventional morality, the static, weak, or rigid moral self falls short of a more developed moral sense, judgment, and motivation needed to live effectively in a constantly changing world.

As individuals and as a society, people are showing signs of "moral blindness" in how they perceive, understand, and objectively grasp existential truth and reality in the moral realm to achieve self-fulfillment goals. There is a strong need for nuanced moral reasoning, moral sense, moral judgment, and moral motivation to develop relevant self-fulfillment goals, which include the urgency to address and solve moral challenges and problems in our world.

When the weak, rigid, or undeveloped moral self dominates one's identity, it reflects moral reasoning that is unhelpful to the individual, as life evidence demonstrates. In contrast, the evolving, more mature self enables us to grow in moral awareness, assisting practical reasoning in understanding current events and situations. The essential moral rationale for today's times and the psychosocial maturity required by the world depend on deeper insight, intuition, and hard-earned wisdom, which we develop through moral consciousness.

The mature moral self is characterized by the moral rationality of moral consciousness, which differs significantly from moral conscience guided by normative morality. The mature moral self enhances individuals' moral reasoning and their ability to act accordingly, helping them develop higher levels of personhood and recognize empathetic kindness and human solidarity as essential to self-fulfillment.

The developed moral self becomes more important in guiding self-fulfillment goals when a person demonstrates in life the moral principles and skills inspired by a commitment to high ideals, human virtues, the common good, human solidarity, meaningful coexistence, and holistic health. It mainly indicates that the person is free from illusions, delusions, and fantasies about life for self-fulfillment goals.

In the rapidly changing moral landscape of the postmodern world, an other-oriented approach to life is vital for the healthy functioning of the moral self. However, instead, we see a world divided by differences such as idiosyncrasies, race, ethnicity, nationality, social status, and more, along with intense hostility between groups and nations. Without embracing an other-oriented approach to human life, we become a fragile humanity, creating a messy and chaotic world. It reflects a world where self-fulfillment is pursued without moral integrity.

Without a mature moral self, we fail to face the existential reality and the objective truth in the moral world. Every day, people become disconnected from this existential truth, which calls them to grow, change, and act with higher ideals and purposes. When we are not linked to existential truth, we miss crucial insights that show us who we truly are, why we are here, and where we are going in life. This disconnection represents the loss of a soul in a person's life. Restoring the soul should be seen as the highest goal of self-fulfillment and the mark of a morally civilized person.

The Public Moral Self

Social scholars believe that since the start of the postmodern era, the gap between the private moral self and the public one has become more evident. It is widely recognized that people often project a hypocritical public image with a distorted or corrupt moral self. However, life experience also shows that a public moral self exists that cannot be completely hidden from others.

In our world, the painfully destructive and disastrous outcomes of behaviors in modern society reveal a persistent public moral self. The terrible acts, crimes, violence, and evil deeds that happen every day demonstrate a dehumanized humanity. There are always implicit and explicit references to people's depraved and malicious moral self, which overwhelmingly dominates the destruction of modern society.

The public moral self in our time is most evident through the deplorable world order and geopolitical turmoil. There are diabolical events and happenings in the postmodern world that are increasingly distressing to the human psyche. We live in a world with dangerous world leaders, kleptocracies, global bad actors, inhumane oligarchs, unscrupulous politicians, depraved public figures, and unjust national and international policies, disrupting and aggravating our daily lives.

The ongoing geopolitical tensions and conflicts, including calculated wars, ethnic cleansing, genocide, terrorism, social violence, civic unrest, racism, and bigotry, do not receive the critical attention they deserve within the framework of the public moral self. Almost everyone tolerates the inhumane conditions and degraded moral environment in our world caused by the malicious public moral self of spiteful and vicious people.

The current global state of socioeconomic disparities, racism, bigotry, heinous crimes, cruel hostilities among groups, and vicious wars between nations reveals the decline of the public moral self, which is lowering the quality of human life worldwide. While we examine issues like wars, genocides, ethnic cleansing, and other evils from a legal standpoint, we often ignore the problems related to the moral health of those responsible.

Bad actors in our world are indifferent or unaware of the consequences of the rogue public moral self. They pursue personal satisfaction in life without regard for others, society, humanity, or the planet. This is the public moral self at work in the fight for dominance by warring nations, the subjugation of dictators and tyrants seeking political power. It is also reflected in the lifestyles of millionaires and billionaires who ignore the survival needs of the millions living in poverty, in citizens exploiting the weak and powerless, and in the global community's complete neglect of the environmental crises threatening humanity's survival.

On no lesser scale, we sustain the public moral self through daily exposure to corruption by local leaders, public officials, and business entrepreneurs. Every day, we tolerate and deal with disgusting, harmful behaviors and misconduct at schools and workplaces, in neighborhoods and private homes, among community members in places of worship, and even among spouses and life partners.

The public moral self is unraveling in modern society. Each day, the underdeveloped public moral self, which is more common in society, leads to dangerous behaviors toward others. People give in to vile actions, causing devastating ripple effects on the broader world. Today, we struggle to embrace humaneness and to develop virtues like compassion, tolerance, patience, endurance, and generosity. We show weak moral capacity for empathetic friendliness, which could strengthen human bonds and promote solidarity. We live in denial of the need to develop moral clarity and purpose in society.

Many people are unaware of the demonic behavioral tendencies that cause serious harm to others, often beyond repair. More individuals pursue their dreams and ambitions, driven by a tendency toward unethical, opportunistic, harmful, and vicious behaviors. In society, we see more people developing a sense of self that reveals malicious tendencies. Evidence of this is seen in the overcrowding of correctional facilities, mental health institutions, rehabilitation centers, and hospitals. Instead of focusing on developing a mature moral self, today's society tends to pathologize and medicalize the moral self, whether public or private.

In the postmodern world, few people show a desire to develop a holistic self or to commit to improving society's welfare. We lack the motivation to pursue higher ideals and purposes in life. Without this drive, we succumb to harmful psychological influences, destructive emotional states, and abnormal, repulsive behavioral tendencies. We neither understand the behavioral consequences of deeper psycho-emotional processes nor connect poor mental health to a corrupt moral self. We live without a practical sense of shared humanity, avoiding the need to confront our true selves and refusing to engage in or commit to self-growth.

In modern society, we recognize that our capacity for empathy and altruism is limited. Empathy and altruism are not as prevalent in people's daily lives as they were in earlier times. The divisiveness, hostility, and enmity that characterize modern society require a public moral self built on human empathy and sensitivity for positive interaction. More than ever, attitudes of tolerance, compassion, and altruism need to resonate in every conflict around the world. The numerous threats facing humanity today highlight the urgent need to develop a public moral self that demonstrates psychosocial maturity in all human goals and actions. This is crucial for fostering empathetic friendliness that promotes human solidarity and meaningful coexistence.

Ordinary people now believe that the global moral climate threatens humanity's future. Experts and scholars say that humanity appears to be heading toward a catastrophic disaster. There are growing calls from social reformers, climate activists, and moral authority figures that the reckless pursuit of human contentment and self-fulfillment in modern times is creating overwhelming existential crises and dangers. All of this underscores the importance of the public moral self.

The hedonic life orientation replaces a life of virtue with one focused on pleasure, and a life of fantasy replaces a life guided by reason. Today, the public moral self is less aware of each other's human rights and life struggles. We often view another person's life as a means to achieve our own goals. The seriousness of this moral tendency is contributing to the widespread growth of utilitarian individualism in the postmodern world.

Self-delusions and illusions about life consistently weaken the absence of a shared deep moral obligation to one another. It reflects a rigid, fragile, and importantly, corrupt public moral self that undercuts the common good and human solidarity. This public moral self cannot hold up in a changing world. It obscures our moral responsibility for each other's welfare. For us to genuinely care about the well-being and future of humanity, everyone needs to grow in their understanding of the public moral self. This will require no extra effort if people commit to self-improvement, aim for higher levels of personhood, and develop a holistic sense of self.

Today, we face significant challenges with the principle of solidarity in human life. We often overlook the fact that life's fulfillment, happiness, and meaning are closely tied to relationships and depend on the moral self engaging in the public sphere. Our weak moral capacity to improve public life, enhance society's welfare, and build a safer world shows that we are grudgingly accepting shared responsibility in modern society. This reveals the public moral self, which neglects the principles of interdependence and human solidarity.

The pursuit of personal happiness and well-being must always be accompanied by a genuine desire for others to share in it. It requires that each individual's moral self be other-oriented, focusing on the common good and overcoming self-centeredness. Unfortunately, in the postmodern world, people tend to prioritize their own interests and goals more.

The core idea of human health focuses on protecting everyone's freedom and happiness. Today's decline of humanity is primarily attributed to the violation of human rights and civil liberties. This indicates that people lack the moral maturity needed for a shared sense of humanity. Usually, people overlook the moral instinct to care and share in daily life.

Behaviors, both private and public, are crucial determinants of public health. Subtle yet harmful behaviors that violate fundamental human rights can threaten public health in ways that healthcare alone might not fully address. Constantly, a person's moral self-concept should make one focus on protecting human rights. The most fundamental right is to live in freedom, which belongs to everyone—rich and poor, powerful and powerless, sinner and saint.

However, many experts estimate that more than half of humanity's right to live in freedom is being violated. Billions of people worldwide are denied this right. They are enslaved by unfair public policies, held back by unjust social systems, and treated inhumanely by others. The dehumanized individuals in our world reflect the public moral self, hindering society's and humanity's well-being through violations of human rights.

Today, violating, restricting, and impeding human rights and civil liberties is a public health crisis. This aspect of public health is not receiving sufficient attention from either society or healthcare systems. As a result, every day, blatant violations of liberty and happiness, bit by bit, harm the health and well-being of society and humanity.

The brutal actions of chauvinists, extremists, supremacists, fanatics, and despots reveal a monstrous and evil side of public morality, causing serious harm worldwide. It exposes the malevolence that remains unaddressed in the human character of those who believe they belong to the "civilized society" and in those who claim to be part of the "civilized world."

The violation of others' freedom and happiness has led to a widespread moral sickness in modern society. It is a severe public health crisis that does not get the attention it deserves. Today's moral decline shows up as a corrupt, distorted, and malicious public moral character, which significantly damages social life.

For humanity to restore stronger moral health that enables the pursuit of liberty and happiness, which everyone is entitled to, it is crucial to examine the agent that supports this—the public moral self. More people live their lives with a distorted, corrupted, depraved, malicious, or unruly public moral self in society. The ability of the public moral self for other-centeredness declines each day in modern society.

The worldviews shaped by conventional morality tools provide people with the framework for their public moral self. Worldwide, the rejection of objective truth and existential reality is causing ripple effects across nations. This trend has grown to a point that it negatively affects the moral foundation of human life. It forms the public moral self, which is shaking the very core of a stable society and healthy humanity. In modern society, the underdeveloped public moral self in individuals gradually undermines the fundamental pillars of a healthy world—interdependence and human solidarity, meaningful coexistence and justice, freedom and peace, and honor and respect.

Every day, we arbitrarily ignore the historical precedents that shape humanity's current situation and underestimate those that could cause negative consequences in the future. It calls for renewing outdated and irrational moral frameworks within our personal, social, political, and economic systems, which can only happen when we collectively depend on the mature public moral self. Through evolving moral awareness, we can nurture the public moral self that helps us create a new world order based on the pursuit of freedom and happiness for everyone. We can only stay hopeful, determined, and optimistic that this will happen. And it will only occur if we develop higher levels of personhood essential for the psychosocial maturity required in our world.

The greatest tragedy of our postmodern era is the lack of trust among people. It stems from behaviors shaped by the public moral self. Without fundamental human trust and solidarity, we can't create a healthier society or a better world for everyone.

In our era, the decline of public trust is evident not only in people's fear and suspicion of others but also in their decreasing confidence in national and international leaders and institutions. This is demonstrated by the 2023 Gallup poll, which tracks the decline from 1979 to 2023 in Americans' confidence in the Supreme Court, Congress, the news media, the church/religion, the military, banks, public schools, big business, and organized labor.[26] The public's loss of faith in social, national, and international institutions is a complex and challenging global issue that shapes how we collectively move toward the future.

What can we learn from people's public moral self that is expressed in our world today?

The answer lies in examining and assessing the behaviors of public figures. Society's well-being is significantly shaped by those who guide its direction. In our world, paying closer attention to the actions of politicians, religious leaders, social celebrities, local community leaders, and other public figures is essential if we want to understand our own moral identity. The public moral self of individuals in high positions is more impressionable than we often realize.

We live in a world where "tell-all" books reveal the moral character of public figures more than ever before. Media reports often highlight actions and behaviors that show more negative than positive aspects of these figures' moral character. It is impossible to ignore the moral reality of society's "leading lights" and high-profile members, whether they are policymakers, politicians, religious

---

[26] Gallup Website, Political Report on 6, 2023

leaders, celebrities, or others who significantly influence society morally. We should recognize how the moral standing of society's pillars shapes our understanding of what it means to be human today.

In today's society, the public's view of the moral character of powerful and influential individuals is concerning. People criticize their depraved, contemptible, and wicked actions, which lead to harmful, life-changing consequences. Social critics strongly argue that the moral character of many public figures today damages society. They firmly claim that many of these figures are even harming the moral fabric of the general population.

We live in a world where the rhetoric of public figures influences everyday people's ideas, opinions, and worldviews. In daily life, public figures affect the moral emotions, thinking, motivation, and behaviors of ordinary people. We often mirror the moral selves of public figures more than we realize. Without us knowing it, or that they are doing it to us, we are held captive by the corrupt and harmful moral selves of public figures.

The repeated dissonance between what politicians and other key figures in society say and do often exposes their corrupt and twisted moral core. Yet, we tend to ignore or overlook the corrupt and depraved morals of policymakers, politicians, religious leaders, and social celebrities. Our submission and compliance toward society's influential members make their character flaws less noticeable. Usually, people are blinded by public status and cannot evaluate morals in real time.

We live in a society where people's critical thinking skills are declining. We often hesitate to judge respected and influential members of society, assuming they are good people. Naivety makes people gullible to those who are prominent and hold social power. The philosopher Descartes warned: to understand what people honestly think, observe what they do rather than what they say.

The depiction of public figures' moral character sets the overall tone for society's moral standards. It acts as a resource that shapes ordinary people's moral ideas, beliefs, attitudes, values, priorities, motivations, and behaviors, thereby influencing society as a whole. The strong influence of the "leading lights" in society is a force worth recognizing for its effect on an individual's public moral sense.

In a sense, the imprints of the moral self of politicians, policymakers, religious leaders, and social celebrities are society's most important vehicles for shaping the public moral self within the general population. People who display a public moral self that harms society are often influenced by the vested interests of public figures. They reveal a moral motivation that aligns with the personal agendas of unscrupulous leaders, some of whom are even blatantly mentally and emotionally unwell.

In today's world, political, religious, and public leaders often act generously and selflessly, but they only pretend to have a mature moral character. However, this conflicts with their actual actions and behaviors. Disgusting and repulsive behaviors and traits expose complete moral corruption. Every day, inflammatory rhetoric and inconsistent actions reveal what the public moral self truly does in our world. More often than not, the moral perception of public figures reflects what one's own public moral self might seem like to others.

We survive through the daily choices, decisions, and actions of many politicians, public figures, civil servants, and religious leaders, which cause instability in society and create chaos in the world. The moral image they display in public service shows they do more harm than good to the moral fabric of society, and indeed, humanity. Evidence from life shows that millions must endure poverty, inhumane living conditions, and a life of endless suffering caused by what public officials and society's prominent figures do or fail to do.

The ongoing toxic influence of corrupt politicians, fanatical religious leaders, and hypocritical celebrities on the world stage never ceases. Their distorted sense of self exposes an incurable, malignant moral core. In many subtle ways, global peace and prosperity face grave threats from public figures. The moral qualities, attitudes, and tendencies they display mostly reveal what is odious, roguish, unsavory, and malevolent. Whether intentionally or not, many public figures today endanger society's moral well-being and humanity as a whole. We must recognize that much of the existential angst in our world is often caused by their actions.

When people fail to pursue objective existential truth, they also neglect to confront the vested interests of public figures who promote division, hatred, and hostility in society. The explicit and covert conspiracy theories in their rhetoric aim to blind and desensitize people to the truth. This rhetoric severely damages the fabric of social trust and human solidarity among ordinary individuals. The distrust caused by the moral posturing of public figures not only gradually harms social welfare and cohesion but also fuels the violent actions of rebel groups and terrorists we face today.

In postmodern times, the moral character of public figures influences people's views, leading to a limited perspective on society's well-being and the future of humanity. Although people are well-informed and rational with science-based knowledge, many public figures continue to have a lasting influence that disrupts social cohesion and weakens the principles of interdependence and human solidarity.

We need to pay closer attention to the moral self and moral health, particularly focusing on the mental health of politicians, religious leaders, and social celebrities who, more than anyone else, often serve as models for society's moral self. In a sense, influential figures in society are the architects of the public moral self, which pollutes the psycho-social environment and fosters a degraded moral climate.

In subtle and unnoticed ways, mentally unstable, morally corrupt, and power-hungry public figures exert the most significant influence on the moral core that shapes society's well-being. A brutal truth for most people to accept is that the degenerate moral character of "leading lights" in society is the primary cause of the corrupt moral climate in the world today.

The corrupt moral self of society's influential members often serves as the leading cause of social disintegration and chaos in our world. Hostility, divisiveness, and social unrest are driven more by the rogue and harmful moral selves of public figures than by any sociocultural influences or factors of postmodern times. People who promote their moral ideals, beliefs, attitudes, and values—even when clear signs of human depravity are evident—nurture an equally rogue and harmful public moral self.

Modern society's health and welfare are more impeded than helped by influential key players. Politicians, policymakers, religious leaders, and other powerful societal figures—such as oil industry tycoons and tech moguls—have the most significant and profound impact on the lives of ordinary people, even if they are often seen as odiously repulsive to the general population.

The harsh reality about our politicians, policymakers, and business leaders is that they lack genuine integrity. In a world where corruption is no longer concealed, the seemingly noble, upright, and gracious public images of these figures often turn out to be just masks for wrongdoing. For the sake of humanity, we must not be fooled by their appearances of decency.

We feel powerless when influential members of society show disdain for the law, violate human rights, and take the innocent hostage. We remain silent in amazement when they buy justice and walk free despite proven crimes. Yet, every day we show respect to public figures who, essentially, negatively affect our well-being and happiness.

We need to be more aware that the public actions of many public figures are often just carefully orchestrated displays of virtue and selflessness in public service. For many, having security details and protection is simply a cover hiding their shocking and disgraceful behaviors. The damaging moral self is masked by the need to be treated as a VIP in society.

We must recognize that the deeply troubling moral environment of today's world arises as much from the moral character of many esteemed, respected, and famous public figures in society as it does from organized criminals, political rebels, and hostile groups who are slandered and seen as outlaws and dishonorable. Understanding that they are equally culpable in wrongdoing is another harsh truth we must confront!

To gauge the influence of the moral character of politicians and policymakers on the broader world, we only need to examine the health and well-being of modern society. Currently, the state of moral health in society is most often reflected in issues such as dehumanizing poverty, social disparities, mental health crises, social violence, heinous crimes, communal conflicts, and many other deplorable acts. Evil behavior has become the new norm for the collective moral self of society.

In our society, we should expect public figures to serve as positive role models of moral integrity rather than simply being socially talented demagogues. It is essential for those seeking public service to demonstrate a higher level of character. They must show the ability to approach public service with a mature moral self, psychological maturity, and foster optimism, mutual respect, and human solidarity among people.

This can only happen if public figures are willing to regularly evaluate their moral selves, which many seem unwilling to do. We rarely see public figures actively engaged in the lifelong process of self-improvement. Usually, most public figures show little interest in achieving higher-level personhood and holistic self-awareness.

Nearly all of society's key players demonstrate the moral quality of a fixed, unchanging, underdeveloped moral self and lack the motivation to grow their moral self and psychosocial maturity. The honor, respect, and deference they are privileged to in society also demand that they develop a mature moral self and the psychosocial maturity necessary in our times.

We cannot improve the world and the future of humanity without influential figures in society becoming positive role models of a mature public moral self. For this to happen, they must demonstrate higher-order personhood through their roles, duties, and obligations to people. Those holding public office need to focus on high-mindedness and noble service. The key mental qualities of people in public service should be assessed through insightfulness, intuitiveness, and perceptiveness, rather than merely compliance with institutional moral standards.

Social scholars argue that a strong moral self is a key resource for public officials, as it can boost their psychological and mental well-being in the workplace, which many seem to need.[27] Failing to work on improving one's moral character is a breach of duty, especially if that character becomes corrupt, depraved, or dishonest. It should be considered a public health crisis when elected officials and public figures jeopardize society and humanity with a rogue, corrupt, or malicious moral self.

Society must urgently focus on prioritizing, emphasizing, and standardizing the moral integrity of public officials, especially our politicians, civil servants, lawmakers, and law enforcement officers. Improving humanity's future depends on holding public figures to the highest human standards as morally mature and responsible individuals in this complex world.

---

[27] Bolino, M. C. & Grant, A. M. The bright side of being prosocial at work, and the dark side, too: a review and agenda for research on other-oriented motives, behavior, and impact in organizations. Academy of Management Annals (Vol.10); 2016

HOW MORAL SELF DEVELOPS IN OUR PERSONHOOD

The chaos in the world reflects humanity's moral health and the moral climate we live in. The news reveals that even those who aim to improve the world can sometimes act in ways that harm society and humanity. It highlights the difference between a fixed, unchanging moral self and a more mature, evolving moral self.

We all want to see a more humane, high-minded, and transparent person in ourselves and others. However, we also tend to cling to the quirks of our moral self, which is shaped by conventional morality. As a result, we live with moral conflicts and dilemmas. We have moral reservations and hesitate to take the stance that would allow us to speak out against what is wrong, unjust, or evil. We remain unaware of our wrongdoings, evil actions, and harmful behaviors, even those occurring around us.

In modern society, human refinement often involves engaging in social interactions with politeness, whether we genuinely agree with others or not. We adopt behaviors to appear cultured, not out of moral conviction. We follow society's moral standards mainly to maintain appearances, not because we genuinely feel morally responsible. These societal expectations for moral image allow us to feign true moral character. As a result, modern society is filled with superficial saints, hypocrites, pretenders, impostors, con artists, and insincere individuals.

When we begin to understand what human life can be like in a society with better levels of moral health, we then value the more developed, mature moral self in ourselves and others. We recognize the need for higher-order personhood to improve everyday attitudes, priorities, and behaviors. We also expect ourselves and others, especially those who play a public role in society, to engage in life with the moral rationality that meets the standards of a mature moral self and supports the welfare and health of society.

We generally do not consider the moral self of personhood as the foundation of human life and existence, the cornerstone. We overlook the moral self that underpins the formation of relationships that are consequential to the world. We ignore the implications of the moral self for society and the world. We devalue the moral self as the behavioral root of everything we do and don't do, which affects humanity and the planet.

Individual and collective moral health depends on the moral self, which is complex and central to moral well-being. It influences not only personal wellness but also the health of humanity and the planet. Our daily actions, relationships, dreams, and aspirations subtly shape societal moral conditions. The moral self acts as a tool that can either build or harm the moral environment worldwide.

The moral climate of our world can be understood and significantly improved through the idea of the moral self. In today's social and cultural environment, although the desire for a more developed and mature moral self to build a better world and ensure the well-being of humanity might seem ambitious, it remains a powerful force for both individual and collective moral well-being, fostering a safer and healthier world.

Both moral conscience and moral consciousness form the foundation of an individual's patterns of thought, feelings, and behavior related to moral health. Usually, people focus on the moral self mainly to appease their moral conscience. This conscience often judges actions against conventional moral standards, acting as a "watchdog" rather than as a tool of true higher-personhood. Life experience shows that, more often than not, this approach only creates an image of morality without fostering the actual moral responses needed in the moment or the moral skills required for current challenges.

Almost everyone tries to appear decent, moral, and in good standing with society. We aim to project an image of moral responsibility. We meet moral standards and fulfill our moral obligations to avoid judgment and condemnation. The moral reasoning and motivation of an average person are driven by fear, shame, and guilt. We develop moral goals mainly to avoid blame, judgment, and internal stress.

However, when someone's moral self is limited to simply meeting the standards of conventional morality, it hampers the moral capacity needed to address more urgent moral problems and dilemmas. It hinders the understanding of objective existential truth, which is necessary for developing deeper moral reasoning, motivation, and responsibility. As a result, people often overlook the significance of higher-order personhood in their daily lives.

The moral self of personhood serves as our primary resource for pursuing higher ideals and discovering more profound meaning and purpose in life. This moral self is mainly shaped by moral consciousness, not moral conscience. It arises from being attuned to objective truth and the existential reality within the moral realm, rather than being blinded by moral utopia or limited by moral boundaries. The confines of conventional moral ideas and rationality restrict a person's moral conscience. In contrast, moral consciousness urges us to go beyond and above the demands of conscience.

Moral consciousness develops a more effective and mature moral self. This moral self is guided by the goals of higher-order personhood, emphasizing otherness and the common good. It fosters moral rationality, encouraging an internalized morality within the individualized moral self. Institutional moral frameworks or bureaucratic truths do not limit this moral rationality. Instead, it incorporates global perspectives to address moral issues. It exemplifies the mature moral self through psychosocial maturity reflected in moral behaviors.

Moral awareness benefits both individuals and society. People who inspire us show a sense of self that grows from moral understanding and higher levels of personhood. This is seen through the mature moral self and psychosocial growth of the individual. The person aims to be deeply human in all life situations.

A genuinely human person who radiates deep contentment and freedom in life exhibits a moral self that isn't burdened by strict moral obligations. Such an individual shines not just by fulfilling moral duties or pursuing moral ideals, but through moral responsibility and appropriately responding to urgent moral issues, challenges, and problems. Those who strive for higher-level personhood become role models for the moral self in society, rather than the prudish or overly scrupulous.

The moral self can either benefit and enrich or ruin and damage one's life and that of others as well. Evidence in life shows that the limits placed on people's moral selves influence both small-scale and large-scale interactions, affecting the health and welfare of individuals, society, and humanity. When people's moral self focuses on egotistical needs, they tend to overlook the common good and the well-being of others.

In our society, many people overlook the fact that taking care of others is a shared moral responsibility that comes with the price of personal happiness, well-being, and good health. Similarly, we often overlook the debt we owe each other in improving society's welfare. The common good and a better world are usually not priorities. It takes a person's mature moral self, guided by moral awareness, for this to happen.

When faced with extraordinary circumstances in the moral realm, moral consciousness supports the moral self, which has a positive impact.

Primarily, moral consciousness allows people to act, achieve, sustain, and affirm the moral self, thereby positively contributing to society's well-being. The postmodern world has introduced new complexities in the social realm, just as it has in the moral sphere, challenging us to develop new skills for human sensitivity and awareness.

The development of one's moral self involves more than just instilling moral values and shaping behavior to enhance relationships. It's also not simply about meeting some standard of human decency. An effective moral self is not solely defined by having a prosocial personality or a tendency toward prosocial actions. Instead, the accurate measure of one's moral self is mainly demonstrated through the ability to resolve moral conflicts and problems, which helps us grow in human solidarity in today's life situations.

This occurs when we directly face the moral challenges in the changing moral landscape of the postmodern world. It requires us to have moral clarity and purpose in modern times. It must be expressed through moral reasoning that is not limited by institutional moral norms, psychosocial maturity, or higher levels of personhood. The effective moral self in the postmodern world must encourage thinking, feeling, and behaviors that promote the well-being of all members of society. Its goal should be to restore humanity's moral health and improve the moral environment worldwide.

The mature moral self develops in individuals only when influenced by moral consciousness, which also benefits society as a whole. Moral consciousness comes from engaging in self-improvement and personal growth. As a lifelong journey, self-improvement is essential for nurturing a mature moral self. In the evolving and complex moral landscape of the postmodern world, traditional morality often serves as a barrier to developing a mature moral self. However, when people are open to change and willing to grow, they see the limitations that traditional morality imposes on the moral self and strive to undergo self-evolution.

The level of a person's moral awareness is fundamental to human consciousness, which neuroscience shows is influenced by brain mechanisms. Developing our moral capacities involves unlocking the innate potential of human nature rather than merely cultivating moral values and ideals of conventional morality. The moral self, emerging from moral consciousness, is a "presentist" phenomenon influenced by brain functions at the moment. It does not imply that it is separate from the immediate moral phenomena and challenges, unlike when the moral self is based on principles and ideals of conventional morality.

Neuroscience reveals that there is an inherent brain network and mechanism for moral reasoning and moral emotion that guide human sensitivity, motivation, and behavior within the moral domain. It is now understood that people's neural abilities are the most crucial in shaping how the moral self manifests in life. Moral capacities are not just measured by simply following moral conscience but by how well one understands the moral entity, which results from moral consciousness.

What modern science shows us is that a person's moral abilities are influenced by human neurobiology. The Science of Neuromorality emphasizes that brain mechanisms are essential for developing moral capacities. It suggests that the moral framework of the moral self can be changed and improved through moral awareness. As we grow in moral consciousness, the moral self becomes significantly different from the one shaped by traditional morality.

Researchers have provided evidence that complex interactions within the brain network directly influence human consciousness; therefore, moral consciousness arises from brain mechanisms.[28] There are specific brain mechanisms dedicated to higher cognitive functions that enable humans to perform intuitive reasoning and objective analysis in the moral realm. These

---

[28] Blumenfeld, H. Brain mechanisms of conscious awareness: detect, pulse, switch and wave. Sage Journals (Vol. 29); 2021

mechanisms can adapt to positively influence people's higher mental abilities and stimulate the primary moral emotion of empathy, which characterizes the capabilities of the mature moral self.

We can only objectively understand matters in the moral domain through brain mechanisms that support higher cognitive functions and moral emotions. The acute awareness of the human mind to grasp the truth and reality of each current moment depends on brain mechanisms for advanced cognitive functioning. Similarly, the relevant moral response to a moral entity is influenced by the brain region that affects empathy capacity and level.

Neuroscience provides neurobiological evidence for moral reasoning, moral sense, moral motivation, and moral behavior in humans.[29] The neuromoral resources of human nature can significantly shape the development of moral identity and the moral self, different from how it develops through traditional morality. The brain's mechanisms of moral consciousness support the objectivity, rationality, and empathetic understanding of the mature moral self. Moral conscience forms the foundation for the limits of objectivity and moral rationality, guided by the dos and don'ts of conventional morality.

As humans, we possess neurobiological resources that can help us rebuild moral identity, recover our moral self, and develop a mature moral and psychosocial self. The regenerative design of moral identity depends on higher cognitive and emotional abilities and functioning. Moral consciousness offers the intuitive, perceptive, and emotional skills necessary for the regenerative process of moral identity.

How people position their moral self in daily attitudes, values, and behaviors determines whether they see it as static and rigid or evolved and mature. The moral self, shaped by normative morality, usually helps protect problematic behaviors and appears moral by meeting expectations and human

---

[29] Robertson D, et.al. The neural processings of moral sensitivity to issues of justice and care. Neuropsycholgia. (2007)

decency. However, it is the mature moral self, which develops through moral consciousness, that is more effective in handling moral conflicts and urgent moral issues.

The mature moral self results from an individual's deeper awareness and perceptions, which help develop broad global perspectives in the moral realm. It surpasses mere moral ideals and principles. The individual's higher cognitive and emotional functions strengthen the moral rationality of the internalized morality of the mature moral self. This is reflected in the psychosocial maturity of higher-order personhood. Higher-order personhood maintains a comprehensive focus on the complexities of the moral domain and is not limited by boundaries in moral reasoning and motivation.

A key aspect of the mature moral self is moral reasoning that significantly differs from the typical moral rationality of conventional morality, which can be unbalanced and problematic in many life situations. It characterizes the internalized morality of the individualizing moral self, rather than the morality of a socially binding one. To effectively address the moral dilemmas and challenges of the postmodern world, a mature moral self is more necessary and relevant in the evolving moral landscape.

Internalized morality provides moral clarity and purpose, which are better suited for a mature moral self. It activates the innate mental capacity for moral reasoning and motivation in the present moment, improving moral responses and behaviors that are relevant and effective. A person's internalized morality evaluates the immediate moral situation differently from conventional morality. This form of morality is not limited by strict right-and-wrong boundaries, unlike traditional morality that emphasizes rigid rules.

The moral self, whether originating from moral consciousness or moral conscience, consistently plays a significant role in shaping individual and collective moral health throughout life and across various cultural contexts. Human awareness levels influence moral understanding, supporting the growth of a mature moral self. During life's journey, an individual's moral self can either promote or hinder the improvement of their personal moral health and the overall moral environment worldwide.

To improve humanity's moral well-being and foster a healthier moral environment worldwide, we need to focus on developing a moral self through moral awareness rather than adhering to the one shaped by traditional morality. The abstract ideals of our outdated moral culture create narrow perspectives that prevent the moral self from effectively resolving conflicts, navigating dilemmas, and addressing urgent moral challenges and issues.

The effective development of humanity's moral health and transforming the moral climate worldwide require us to focus on the moral self that stems from moral consciousness. It is people's moral consciousness that helps evaluate specific positive and negative moral phenomena within the moral realm. The appropriate moral response to urgent, current moral issues depends on moral consciousness, not on moral ideals, principles, or norms. When a person is "morally awakened and charged" by moral consciousness, they are not bound by old familiar moral recipes but instead understand and judge moral phenomena through comprehensive perspectives and respond to pressing moral issues in a more relevant way.

The practical ways we develop the moral self of personhood include (1) striving for higher-order personhood, (2) enriching one's working self-concept and self-identity, and (3) cultivating a sense of aesthetics in human life.

Pursuing Higher-Order Personhood

Evidence from life demonstrates that people in modern society often have an unstable sense of self and a troubling identity. Many see this as a result of the socially influenced moral self. Most individuals display a moral self connected to conventional morals. They aim to think and act in ways that only give the illusion of being morally upright and responsible, rather than honestly confronting or resolving critical moral issues.

At the same time, it is also evident in society that the moral self people adopt fosters guilt, self-hatred, remorse, fear, and other negative feelings, leading to psycho-emotional and psychosocial instability, and even worsening underlying mental health issues. The chaos and turmoil in our individual lives, society, and the world indicate that we are not developing the mature moral self of higher-level personhood.

This suggests that modern society often fails to recognize the vital role of higher-order personhood in human life. We tend to prioritize face-saving motives of the moral self over authentic self-growth. Few realize how essential higher-order personhood and a mature moral self are for improving personal happiness, well-being, and societal progress. Experience shows that the moral self can either positively or negatively affect our humanity and influence society's overall well-being.

In the moral landscape of the postmodern world, moral conscience influences individuals' cognitive, psycho-emotional, and psychosocial processes in different ways from moral consciousness. Evidence from life shows that people often display thinking, emotional, and behavioral patterns that can be harmful to themselves and those around them. The many adverse effects of these tendencies in society highlight the inadequate regulatory skills of the moral self.

Our sense of who we are as humans is shaped mainly by how we respond to moral issues in life. Simply feeling guilty after wrongdoing or showing remorse and making amends for harm caused to others reflects a kind of moral self that is judged by conventional morality, not higher-level personhood. In contrast, when we think about developing the moral self through higher-level personhood, there is no room for harming or hurting others—only for caring, nurturing, and protecting. The moral self aims for empathetic friendliness, human solidarity, and the common good.

People rarely assess harmful and dangerous behaviors that negatively impact society's health and well-being to understand how they reflect human nature in our world. Few recognize the role of the moral self in defining what it means to be human. Evidence from life suggests that, for many, this leads to a confused, troubled, and delusional sense of self. The disintegration and incoherence of the self, in terms of selfhood, indicate a fragmented sense of personhood.

We need a concept of personhood that embodies human virtues, nobility, and otherness. Higher-order personhood is an organic human structure that develops naturally over time.[30] It cannot be feigned, improvised at will, or achieved instantly. We grow into higher-order personhood by prioritizing moral identity and moral self as essential to human transformation.

Higher-order personhood develops through self-evolution. It is a worthwhile goal in the pursuit of self-fulfillment. It provides a more profound sense of fulfillment than any other experience. Self-evolution is mainly driven by the expansion of human consciousness within an individual. This consciousness improves self-awareness, perception, insight, intuition, and emotional skills like empathy, sensitivity, and tenderness, which enhance a person's inner growth and psychosocial maturity.

Human consciousness plays a vital role throughout life in shaping our identity, how we live, and what we're meant to achieve. We operate based on either a fixed or a changing human consciousness. The moral realm is closely linked to human consciousness. As one's consciousness develops, it gradually involves the individual gaining moral awareness and psycho-emotional clarity for better moral reasoning, understanding, and motivation.

Neuroscience indicates that human consciousness originates from brain processes within an individual.[31] Through moral awareness, the human

---

[30] Lau, H. and Rosenthal, D. Empirical Support for Higher-Order Theories of Conscious Awareness. Trends in Cognitive Sciences (Vol. 15); 2011.
[31] Lau, H. and Rosenthal, D. Empirical Support for Higher-Order Theories of Conscious Awareness. Trends in Cognitive Sciences (Vol. 15); 2011.

brain can help us grow, develop, and strengthen our internal morals in ways that go beyond traditional morality. Neuroscience reveals that forming a mature moral self involves a complex interaction of a person's genetic, neurobiological, and socio-cultural factors, along with patterns of self-evolution. Importantly, this also places the moral self within the neurobiological condition of individuals.

People's moral awareness is closely connected to their overall human consciousness. Life experiences demonstrate that moral awareness influences moral reasoning and actions beyond simply following norms, rules, or laws. A mature moral self emerges from this moral awareness, which mainly results from self-evolution driven by the expansion of human consciousness. Scholars agree that levels of human consciousness shape moral awareness in individuals.[32]

The emancipated moral self mainly results from moral consciousness. As human consciousness develops, it leads to a mature moral self and psychosocial maturity, which represent higher levels of personhood. Conversely, the rigid moral self, often seen in daily life, provides predetermined and repetitive responses during moral crises and is rooted in static human consciousness.

Higher-order personhood is more connected to moral awareness than to moral conscience. As individuals progress to higher levels of human consciousness, they become less limited by strict moral ideals and principles. Their moral reasoning extends beyond institutional norms, and their motivations and actions are not confined by rigid morality. Psychosocial maturity represents an internalized morality that influences their life choices.

Higher-order personhood is essential for developing a mature moral identity and the psychosocial maturity needed in postmodern times. It is vital

---

[32] Levy, N. Consciousness and Moral Responsibility. Oxford University Press; 2014.
Levy N. The Value of Consciousness. Journal of Consciousness Studies; January, 2014

to nurture and deepen our empathetic kindness toward others. The effort to be human in our world highlights that developing higher-order personhood occurs gradually through a lifelong process of self-evolution that shapes the mature moral self.

When positive changes happen in our sense of personhood, they help improve society's well-being. The mature moral self of personhood is essential to how we define humanity in the postmodern world. This mature moral self supports everyday moral actions, which in turn boost the health and well-being of society. These actions come from empathetic friendliness that develops from the psychosocial maturity of higher-level personhood.

The mature moral self is best reflected in the behaviors of higher-order personhood through the way we live. Moral consciousness consistently helps the mature moral self to sustain itself individually. There are steady and reliable positive responses to urgent moral issues. In contrast, the rules of conventional morality limit the reactions of a static, unchanging moral self.

Higher-order personhood underpins the development of comprehensive global perspectives on life, especially amid a constantly shifting moral landscape. It shapes how we interpret, assign meaning to, and value everyday moral events. It encourages uncommon moral responses when facing dilemmas. It promotes a dynamic moral self that reacts differently to moral issues and challenges compared to lower-order personhood.

When we develop the ability to see everyone as deserving of human respect, dignity, and care, we think, feel, and act from a higher sense of personhood. This is evident in the moral reasoning of a mature moral self and the psychosocial growth of an individual. Higher-order personhood allows people to engage positively in life through moral capacities that support one another. The moral skills and attitudes used when relating to others differ from those of someone who is simply following moral rules.

The mature moral self is essential for guiding our behavior toward others. It consistently strives to develop a relational working self-concept and self-identity, focusing on how we treat others. The moral framework of the mature self benefits an individual's psycho-emotional and behavioral qualities, helping to enhance and strengthen relationships. It manifests through psycho-social maturity, resilience, integrity, and character, which define a higher level of personhood.

When it comes to fundamental human dignity and the rights of others, moral consciousness helps better assess whether entities are morally positive or negative. A person's moral consciousness allows them to modify the psycho-emotional process of the moral self, which enhances moral sensitivity, awareness, and enriches human relationships. Conversely, moral conscience limits psychosocial feelings, values, and attitudes through moral imperatives and ideals. A static, rigid moral self prevents a person from developing broader perspectives in the moral realm.

People's moral framework can influence whether we respect or despise human dignity and the natural rights that stem from it. History shows that conventional morality often allows the moral self within individuals to violate human dignity and rights. The moral framework does not prevent behaviors with a rigid, unchanging moral self, even when there is a "working conscience" in people.

Respecting human dignity in all situations requires more than just following prescribed morality. It also involves accepting moral responsibility for the well-being of others, regardless of who they are. Moral awareness is a more effective resource than moral conscience for developing thinking, emotional responses, and behaviors that foster positive relationships.

In postmodern times, higher-order personhood, which is the hallmark of a genuinely human individual, reflects the moral identity and moral self that are distinctly shaped by advanced cognitive functions and empathetic abilities. Neuroscience provides evidence of neural mechanisms involved in human development and the growth of a person. The neurobiological basis for the mature moral self, psychosocial maturity, and higher-order personhood highlights that more than just conventional morality is required to be considered a human person.

Central to higher-order personhood are the regenerative design of moral identity and the rehabilitation of the moral self. It appears in the mature moral self as an individualizing moral self, rather than a socially bonding one. Today's social and cultural changes require people to commit to self-evolution to develop the mature moral self and the psychosocial maturity needed in the world. Self-evolution primarily reestablishes moral identity and restores the moral self, focusing on the individualizing moral self.

The moral identity and moral self that meet the criteria for moral agency of higher-order personhood in the postmodern world should primarily be driven by moral concern and responsibility rooted in the principles of interdependence, human solidarity, and shared humanity. These elements of the moral sphere in human life are better guided by moral consciousness than by normative morality and the institutional pursuit of truth.

Personhood development is a lifelong journey. In modern times, developing higher-level personhood aims to foster appropriate and effective moral thinking and behaviors. In our constantly changing and challenging moral environment, living with meaning and purpose requires us to strive for a mature moral self and psychosocial maturity. We are called to renew our moral identity and rebuild the moral self as ongoing elements that promote higher-order personhood to strengthen human qualities and humane capabilities. The mature moral self supports the development of moral concern, sensitivity, and sensibility, which go beyond moral conventions and normative rules, to define higher-order personhood. We are encouraged to cultivate moral health as a crucial aspect of well-being if we want to experience a higher form of humanity in our morally complex world.

There is a linear progression in the development of a person's moral self. This resembles how our primitive ancestors shifted from a basic existence to a more advanced one. In today's world, the growth of our moral self alone gives us the psychological, emotional, and social tools to become less self-centered and more other-focused. This change helps us live in harmony, build human solidarity, and work together for the common good.

Higher-order personhood highlights social integration and cohesion. Developing a healthy sense of personhood equals achieving psychosocial maturity, which is essential for relating to others. This process always involves the innate moral capacities of the individual during interactions. When it occurs, the conflicting implications of the moral self guided by conventional morality are no longer present.

Higher-order personhood in individuals is more often achieved through moral consciousness than by pursuing moral rules and ideals. It is best demonstrated in human sensitivity, sensibility, and appropriate responses to urgent moral issues affecting human life. The sense of personhood that negatively impacts societal welfare, human health, and the moral environment in the world is guided by moral conscience, not moral consciousness.

A healthier society and humanity depend on individuals' higher-level personhood. Commitment to self-improvement, authentic personhood, and holistic selfhood is the most urgent need in this postmodern world for meaningful connections and relationships that support society and mankind. This is the only way to escape decadent, depraved, and unstable personhood and delusional selfhood that are increasingly common and weaken social cohesion and human solidarity. Human maturity is reflected through the moral self in actions that heal and nurture relationships, rather than hurt or harm them.

Enriching One's Working Self-Concept and Self-Identity

All our efforts and relationships as humans are built on the working self-concept and self-identity. As mentioned earlier, these are a person's evolving and context-dependent view of their own personhood. They relate to how one perceives oneself and one's role in the world. The moral self is a crucial part of the working self-concept and self-identity, shaping how one lives.

Our working self-concept and self-identity influence how we behave in moral issues in life. Modern psychology emphasizes that these aspects are essential for our sense of self and impact our health and relationship patterns.[33] To a large degree, they affect society's overall well-being. Social scientists explain that people's working self-concept and self-identity have notable external effects and shape society's overall dynamics.[34]

Everyone's working self-concept and self-identity influence the current moral climate worldwide. In modern society, fleeting, superficial, and unnecessary things dominate people's values, attitudes, and behaviors. The focus on external appearances has made individuals vulnerable to an unstable "psychic world." This mindset aligns with the psycho-emotional processes of people's working self-concept and self-identity, which are marked by a continuous shifting of inner balance, harmony, and stability. Often, people's working self-concept and self-identity show that they feel confused and disoriented in life.

Scholars and experts argue that a person's inner balance and harmony are crucial for fostering human solidarity, global peace, and overall happiness. Today, the impact of people's complex and troubled "psychic world" is evident in feelings of fragmented identity and delusional self-perception. This is reflected in how individuals view themselves, which complicates not only personal lives but also societal well-being.

As noted earlier, the perception of one's moral self is central to the

---

[33] Leary MR & Tangney JP (Editors) Handbook of Self and Identity. Guilford Press (2013)
[34] Hogg, M.A., Self-uncertainty and group identification: Consequences for social identity, group behavior, intergroup relations, and society. Advances in Experimental Social Psychology (Vol. 64); 2021.

working self-concept and self-identity. The behaviors of one's moral self influence the psycho-emotional— the "psychic world"— and social dynamics of the individual. Essentially, the working self-concept and self-identity in today's society most often show that the moral self of personhood neither helps people gain insights into themselves nor enriches human life.

Modern health sciences emphasize that a person's psycho-emotional stability is essential for developing higher-level personhood, which is reflected in the behaviors of a mature moral self and psychosocial maturity. Without these, the working self-concept and self-identity can cause many problems for ourselves and others.

Today, we painfully witness numerous examples of human depravity on the world stage. Every day, we find ourselves suspecting, doubting, and questioning each other's moral integrity. But beyond mere lack or weakness of moral integrity, moral identity plays a crucial role in shaping the moral framework of a person's everyday self-concept and self-identity. Moral identity is fundamental to the moral self, reflecting the core nature of humanity. The compassionate and altruistic tendencies, as well as the cold, hard-hearted, and inhumane traits in people, are connected to their moral identity.

The core personality style and functioning of a person are connected to the psycho-emotional process of moral identity. The moral self, which aligns with moral identity, includes the working self-concept and self-identity within a person's everyday personality style and functioning. The moral self influences moral perceptions, beliefs, attitudes, and the overall understanding of the world within one's working self-concept and self-identity. The typical personality traits of an individual are based on the foundational psycho-emotional processes of moral identity and the behaviors of the moral self.

Therefore, beyond issues such as violations of ethical and moral standards, laws, crimes, violence, corruption, fraud, malfeasance, and other social problems, it is primarily the unresolved issues of moral identity within an individual that impact societal well-being. These unresolved issues damage a person's moral self, their self-concept, and self-identity at work, which can lead to abnormal behaviors that negatively influence the moral environment of society.

The everyday prosocial or antisocial behaviors reveal how moral identity influences and motivates the moral self. The tendency toward virtues, integrity, and other moral qualities, or their opposites, shows how moral identity shapes the moral self within a person's daily self-concept and identity. This moral self affects both individual well-being and societal health through self-perception and self-identity.

Regarding the working self-concept and self-identity, it's important to weigh the advantages and disadvantages of moral identity. It shapes the moral self, which influences daily thoughts, feelings, and actions, affecting the working self-concept and self-identity that are demonstrated each day in the moral sphere.

The unresolved issues of moral identity are at the root of all suffering and harm to oneself and others. They form the foundation of the moral self, which fosters a corrupt moral environment in society. The dishonest, spiteful, and vicious elements within people's working self-concept and self-identity are some of the greatest threats of our time. This moral self, central to modern human struggles, problems, and evils, is a core issue. Human life and existence depend on this fragile moral self.

Typically, people's moral self is shaped by moral systems. Someone who follows conventional morality develops specific ways of thinking and behavior patterns linked to their moral self and adopts these patterns. This moral self is a crucial part of how people see and define themselves at work. A major problem with this moral self is the limitations it places on people's self-view and self-identity in the workplace. The moral abilities and reasoning tied to the self-concept and self-identity at work are restricted, which limits broader, global perspectives in moral understanding.

A static, rigid, undeveloped moral self limits a person's moral understanding, reasoning, motivation, and actions to their daily self-concept and identity. Furthermore, as life evidence shows, the strongly established static, rigid, or undeveloped moral self of individuals is often driven by fleeting desires, face-saving aims, and self-centered goals rather than the common good, societal welfare, or human solidarity.

People's working self-concept and self-identity are essential in shaping how they think, behave, and relate in daily life. The idea of one's moral self, typically rooted in society's moral culture, conventions, and traditions, is beginning to weaken the version that is more relevant for the working self-concept and self-identity today. When the moral self undermines higher ideals and life goals of the working self-concept and self-identity, it gradually leads to a decline in moral standards worldwide.

Experts argue that traditional morality blocks individuals' working self-concept and self-identity when facing moral challenges today.[35] They highlight that these aspects of the self significantly influence societal health and well-being, and this effect is inevitable. Daily behaviors observed in modern society serve as evidence of people's working self-concept and self-identity, which are driven by stronger self-centered values and priorities, reflecting a decreased capacity for other-centeredness in people's lifestyles.

Besides the traditional morality's impact on the fixed, strict moral self associated with the working self-concept and self-identity, another concern involves social and cultural influences on the moral self. When moral identity aligns with social and cultural factors, the moral self tends to reflect the generalized version. Today's sociocultural influences shaping people's moral identity are fostering a more flexible moral self that influences their daily work

---

[35] Cui, P. et.al. Moral identity and subjective well-being: The mediating role of identity commitment quality. Int. J. Res Public Health (Vol. 18); 2021

self-concept and self-identity.

In our era, the global cultural phenomena of consumerism, individualism, and hedonism are negatively impacting people's working self-concept and self-identity. The moral self within these aspects aligns with the prevailing moral reasoning and behaviors in the sociocultural environment. As life evidence shows, the subsequent moral sense, motivation, and behavior of people's moral self are driven by ego needs, insatiable desires, and hedonic tendencies.

Cultural critics argue that the moral framework of modern society is built on self-deception and illusions of self-fulfillment. Typically, people's moral self aligns with a system shaped by social and cultural influences. The moral self rooted in this framework connects with individuals' working self-concept and self-identity. Most people remain stuck in a static moral self concerning their working self-concept and self-identity.

Many people overlook how harmful influences from sociocultural factors affect modern society, which underpin issues related to moral identity and the moral self. When the moral self is held hostage to illusions and delusions, a person's working self-concept and self-identity are negatively affected, impacting their way of life and mode of existence. Today, we understand that people's working self-concept and self-identity can lead to abnormal, harmful, and dangerous behaviors that spread throughout modern life. These behaviors not only damage individuals' reputations but also impose significant socioeconomic costs on society as a whole.

In postmodern times, people's daily thoughts and behaviors are not strongly motivated by the principles of interdependence, human solidarity, and coexistence. This shows that their working self-concept and self-identity are less shaped by the mature moral self. Not everyone finds the motivation to develop or nurture the mature moral self that benefits their working self-concept and self-identity.

People generally show little interest in putting in the effort needed for self-improvement in a constantly changing world. We often resist change and avoid challenges that could enhance our working self-concept and self-identity, which would, in turn, improve the quality of human life for everyone. However, paying closer attention to the working self-concept and self-identity is crucial if we want to regenerate moral identity, rebuild the moral self, and develop higher levels of personhood.

Every day, we develop perceptions of ourselves, and others form perceptions of us through the working self-concept and self-identity. These perceptions of personhood are mainly reflected in behaviors linked to the working self-concept and self-identity, especially in the moral realm. Such perceptions impact our sense of self and affect society's overall well-being. How we see ourselves and how others perceive us can either reinforce or weaken our active personhood and self-awareness, which, in turn, shape the world we create each day through our actions and behaviors via the working self-concept and self-identity.

The subjective perceptions of behavioral and relational patterns reveal the strengths and weaknesses of the working self-concept and self-identity, which include moral identity and moral self. When subjective perceptions of the working self-concept and self-identity do not align with others' perceptions, it often indicates issues related to integrity, character, self-centeredness, and the challenge of being other-focused. Conversely, positive subjective perceptions provide the experience of a well-developed moral self, higher-order personhood, and a full sense of selfhood.

Most people are aware of the "actual self" and the "ideal self," but not of the "real self" of personhood. The "actual self" is how they currently see themselves in their working self-concept and self-identity, while the "ideal self" is who they hope or wish to be within the same self-concept. Notably, the real self fulfills the psychosocial need for consistency in personhood, which appears in people's working self-concept and self-identity.

It should be emphasized that the ideal self someone desires in their working self-concept and self-identity is either the ideal self they want to become or the one they believe others expect and/or perceive them to have. When the "ideal self" is driven by what a person thinks others see as ideal or expect from them, they may become more disconnected from their true self. We often misunderstand who we truly are when we try to meet others' expectations of how they want us to behave. To fulfill these expectations, we adopt the roles they imagine we should play.

The actual self and the ideal self differ from a person's true self. Life experiences show that the true self is often hard for others to see and difficult for us to recognize in ourselves. Today, we often notice that a person's true self is very different from both their actual self and their ideal self. When people aim for higher moral standards, they are working to align with their true self.

Those who value staying true to their authentic selves are driven to develop their moral character through self-growth. It is only when a person recognizes and accepts their true self, and differentiates between their real, actual, and ideal selves, that they engage in the process of self-evolution. At the heart of a mature moral self, psychosocial maturity, personal health, and well-being are always grounded in the true self; meanwhile, the pseudo-self leads to various complex issues that affect a person's health and relationships.

In our high-tech world, the actual, ideal, and real selves—separated by our working self-concept and self-identity—must be considered in the context of the internet. There is a dynamic interaction between people's self-structure components and digital devices. Often, without realizing it, the working self-concept and self-identity people develop are influenced by the intensity of online influencers and the powerful forces of media content.

Today, people define who they are based on online influences and media content. Internet culture increasingly links individuals' self-understanding to these online influences and media. This also means that, for many, the real self and pseudo-self are often indistinguishable in the postmodern world. In real-life situations, the working self-concept and self-identity shaped by internet culture cause individuals to experience a blurred sense of personhood. The "real me" feels disconnected from one's sense of self, and there is only an apparent "real me."

Bad actors online and in the media create problems for people by making it difficult to distinguish their true self from their pseudo-self within their work self-concept and self-identity. The personhood anomalies of bad actors distort and overshadow the superficial self-concept and self-identity that people internalize. The negative influence of the fraudulent selfhood of online strangers produces psycho-emotional conditions that often harm people's sense of self. In modern society, the sense of pseudo-self dominates the work self-concept and self-identity, which negatively affects logical thinking for moral reasoning and motivates appropriate public behaviors. The moral sense and motivation guiding daily actions often imitate the moral self of strangers.

The digital world has a greater negative impact on people's working self-concept and self-identity than most realize. These aspects, which influence daily actions, often increase the effect of dishonest and questionable strangers encountered online who exhibit a corrupt moral self. In a highly connected society, how individuals' moral self combines with their working self-concept and self-identity reflects how media personalities and online influencers portray moral selves. This should raise concerns about the risks that online interactions and media influence pose to one's working self-concept and self-identity.

We often believe we have some control and choice in our online interactions with others. However, in reality, our moral self is constantly challenged within our working self-concept and self-identity. Frequently, we adopt a moral self of personhood that is less than what we might truly possess, which typically benefits our working self-concept and self-identity. Today, it is common for us to resist, in a defiant manner, the moral self of our working self-concept and self-identity, even though it already provides us with benefits.

Cultural critics argue that our advanced communication technology has contributed to the loss and denial of objective truth and reality, making the true self indistinguishable from the pseudo-self. They believe people create a delusional sense of identity and often justify roles they are not or have yet to understand. The critics contend that internet culture has fostered a new human reality, with disastrous effects on what it means to be human today.

When a person intentionally lives true to their authentic self, their moral capacity encourages positive actions. These actions foster favorable perceptions that reflect the integrity of their functional self-concept and self-identity. The degree to which someone values these positive perceptions influences how much the mature moral self helps develop the real self.

In contrast, when we live with the pseudo-self, we often experience psychological tension caused by egregious behavior. It threatens or results in self-disintegration, leading to a problematic working self-concept and self-identity. This is a more common experience of people's self-concept and self-identity in modern society, which symbolizes the "new" human phenomenon in the postmodern world.

When we struggle to consistently think, feel, and behave in accordance with the real self, a pattern of positive outcomes occurs because of the psychological discomfort with our perceptions of selfhood. This discomfort triggers a desire and motivation to maintain a moral self that aligns with the real self. During mental and emotional blockages, the restorative design of moral identity helps rebuild the moral self so it corresponds with the real self within the active self-concept and self-identity. Strengthening the real self outweighs the pseudo-self in the moral realm. The restorative design of moral identity aims to help the moral self align with the real self.

The lack of a self-regulatory mechanism for the internalized moral identity weakens the moral self in terms of selfhood. It results from tolerating dissonance between the real self and the pseudo-self within the working self-concept and self-identity. This ongoing acceptance of dissonance between the real self and the pseudo-self regularly hinders the essential need for self-growth. It blocks the development of higher-order personhood within people's working self-concept and self-identity. Additionally, it undermines the goals of a mature moral self and psychosocial maturity in daily life.

In literature, researchers and experts see the role of "moral cleansing" as essential for counteracting the self-disintegrative tendencies that come from people's thinking and behavior patterns.[36] The working self-concept and self-identity are assessed to help restore internalized moral identity and reshape the moral self.

The purpose of "moral cleansing" is to give an individual a clear understanding of their mature moral self within their work self-concept and self-identity.[37] This mostly helps guide the person toward engaging in positive behaviors. The positive valence of one's internalized moral identity reduces the likelihood of serious negative behaviors. Positive behaviors especially encourage favorable perceptions through the mature moral self embedded in the work self-concept and self-identity.

The concept of "moral cleansing" describes a conscious effort by an individual to address issues in moral identity that underlie harmful behaviors of the moral self. It aims to enhance the psychological and emotional aspects of internalized moral identity. This involves working through self-evolution processes to develop a mature moral self and psychosocial maturity, which reflect higher-level personhood. Such growth benefits the working self-concept

---

[36] Brañas-Garza, P., Bucheli, M., Espinosa, M.P., & García-Muñoz, T. Moral cleansing and moral licenses: Experimental evidence. ESI Working Paper, Chapman University Digital Common; (2011)

[37] Gotowiec S, van Mastrigt S. Having versus doing: The roles of moral identity internalization and symbolization for prosocial behaviors. The Journal of Social Psychology. 2019

and self-identity.

The work involved in "moral cleansing" primarily aims to reshape one's moral self within their working self-concept and self-identity by renewing that moral identity. Researchers have found that "moral cleansing" helps individuals strive to acquire symbols of their true self within the working self-concept and self-identity. Exploring our internalized moral identity directly influences changes in the moral self and perceptions of the true self, helping to develop a working self-concept and self-identity that support daily thoughts and actions. Individuals tend to value having positive perceptions of their true self within the working self-concept and self-identity.

Deliberate efforts to positively symbolize the good aspects of selfhood within the working self-concept and self-identity align with the level of positive behaviors. Without regenerative design for one's moral identity, there is less opportunity to develop positive moral behaviors that reflect the true self within the working self-concept and self-identity.

People's sense of incompleteness when they fail to meet the behavioral performance threshold is crucial for developing a more positive self-concept and self-identity. Moral identity, moral self, and daily behaviors work together to enhance positive perceptions of personhood and foster a more favorable self-view. Modern psychology shows that the working self-concept and self-identity are constantly changing and actively help evaluate the moral self for moral cleansing.[38]

The human desire for positive perceptions of personhood should be the main goal guiding daily actions that aim to enhance the true self within people's working self-concept and self-identity. Behaviors promoted by a mature moral self help develop perceptions of the true self that positively

---

[38] Sachdeva S, et.al. Sinning saints and saintly sinners: the paradox of moral self-regulation. Psychol. Sci. Vol 20 (4); 2009
West C, Zhong CB. Moral Cleansing. Curr Opi Psychol. Vol 6; 2015

influence the working self-concept and self-identity. Conversely, allowing indiscriminate behaviors through a dissolute moral identity harms perceptions of selfhood linked to the working self-concept and self-identity.

A sordid moral identity has many negative effects on a person's moral self within their working self-concept and self-identity. The harmful behaviors that result from it, when repeated over time, further diminish perceptions of the true self within these self-concepts. The unchanging moral identity that influences how the true self is viewed within one's working self-concept and self-identity requires "moral cleansing."

When people assess their working self-concept and self-identity, they also consider any dissonances between the real self and the pseudo-self of personhood. The strength of good and correct moral reasoning, judgments, and behaviors is shown in daily life by experiencing less dissonance within one's selfhood caused by conflicts between the real self and the pseudo-self.

Regarding how moral identity affects the real self within an individual's working self-concept and self-identity, research indicates that moral identity can either positively or negatively influence self-esteem.[39] Self-esteem is a crucial part of the self-concept and self-identity shaped by the moral self. It is an emotional response to the moral self and moral identity that consistently impacts behaviors, which in turn affect perceptions of personhood—either weakening or strengthening the working self-concept and self-identity.

Positive behaviors that boost self-esteem help maintain the true self within the working self-concept and self-identity through the mature moral self. They arise from efforts to rebuild moral identity and restore the moral self. Developing the mature moral self separates the authentic self from the pseudo-self and enhances self-esteem. Modern health sciences suggest that self-esteem

---

[39] Krettenauer T. et.al. Daily moral identity: Linkages with integrity and compassion. Journal of Pers. 90, 2022

plays a vital role in preserving a sense of self that fosters good health, especially holistic health, and societal well-being.[40]

A person's self-esteem and overall sense of self-worth are unlikely to be impacted by occasional mistakes in moral judgment and behavior. However, long-term poor self-esteem and low self-worth result from negative evaluations of oneself. These are influenced by perceptions of moral behavior through the working self-concept and self-identity. The moral self of a person is central to this judgment. To encourage behavioral changes that improve self-esteem, the mature moral self always takes priority over the less developed moral self within the working self-concept and self-identity.

The moral identity guiding a person's moral self predicts their overall self-esteem. It serves as the most crucial tool for boosting self-esteem. Daily actions, which stem directly from the moral self, influence self-esteem either positively or negatively. When self-esteem becomes unstable, a negative moral identity can affect the behavior of the moral self. To stabilize overall self-esteem, it's important to carefully analyze behaviors to understand the moral identity shaping the moral self. When general self-esteem is destabilized, it indicates a need for "moral cleansing."

The assessment of the moral self within the working self-concept and self-identity is driven by the desire to revive moral identity for behavioral improvements. When the real self interacts with the moral identity, a person's behaviors enhance self-esteem. They develop positive perceptions of the mature moral self within their working self-concept and self-identity.

A person's self-esteem influences not only their personal well-being but also the overall health of society. The moral self shapes actions that affect both individual self-esteem and societal well-being. Strong self-esteem is a clear

---

[40] Baumeister RF, et.al. Does self-esteem cause better performance, interpersonal success, happiness, or healthier lifestyles? Psycho Sci (Vol 4); 2003

sign of mental and social health in individuals and indicates a healthy society.

Cultivating the Aesthetic Appreciation of Human Life

Primarily, genuine progress toward a healthier humanity, a shifted moral environment, and a better world depends on our aesthetic appreciation of human life. Aesthetics in life influences people's moral perspectives and motivation. Aesthetic sensibility guides our pursuit of a world that, although never perfect, strives to be as close to an ideal as possible. These pursuits stem from the developed moral core of personhood.

The significance of engaging with the aesthetic sense in human life lies in shaping the right moral rationale, abilities, and attitude. It involves strengthening moral capacities to enhance the quality of life. It also signifies moral motivation that reenergizes us to develop behaviors and relationship patterns that foster human solidarity. Above all, it emphasizes maintaining a unifying focus on the humanity we can become.

Aesthetics in human life is not about beauty or elegance, but about a sense of coherence in vision. It involves bringing together different social, cultural, political, and moral elements to support a healthier humanity and a better world. The polarization we see in humanity today reflects a poor aesthetic sense of human life. Without a unified focus on the kind of humanity we aspire to, we are left to survive in a chaotic and dangerous world.

Central to envisioning a healthier humanity and a better world is the moral health of all peoples and nations. It requires a commitment to self-improvement and the development of a higher sense of personhood for a mature moral self and psychosocial maturity. The idea of coherence to unify humanity depends on us focusing on moral health. Modern health sciences show that with higher levels of moral health, we engage in life fully — utilizing our intellectual, spiritual, and aesthetic capacities![41]

---

[41] Hofmann, B.M. Moral obligations towards human persons' wellbeing versus their suffering: An analysis of perspectives of moral philosophy. Health Policy (Vol. 142); 1924.

Moral health is the key to a complete sense of self, which is vital for building a healthier humanity and a better world. This sense of self is more influential than any imposed theoretical system, ideological utopias, or the noisy chorus of modern dogmatic experts and armchair pundits claiming to improve the world. Most importantly, one's holistic selfhood fuels the appreciation of human life through aesthetics. Without an aesthetic view of human life, our efforts will always fall short of reaching their true potential to foster a healthier humanity and a better world.

The effort to unify humanity starts with cultivating a holistic sense of self within the mature moral individual who is involved in our working self-concept and self-identity. This requires us to change outdated thinking and behavioral patterns and to develop the moral reasoning of a mature moral self to improve psychosocial maturity in human interactions. When this happens, we are guided by higher ideals and purposes to foster the spirit of human solidarity, committed to the moral responsibility of enhancing others' welfare, and always working toward the common good.

We depend on the moral self to support intentional and logical moral reasoning, thereby fostering a healthy humanity and a humane world. This requires the moral self to seek objective truth to bridge individual differences through compromises. In everyday life, only the mature moral self and psychosocial maturity enable a sharp focus on a coherent, vibrant, and unified humanity. It promotes moral sense, reasoning, and motivation in ways that differ from the rigid, static moral self, which is fixated on conforming to conventional morality. The rules and ideals of traditional morality have not created a healthy humanity or a humane world.

It takes a mature moral self to prioritize the well-being of humanity

---

Adamou, M. et.al. The wellbeing thermometer: a novel framework for measuring wellbeing. Psychology (Vol. 11), Scientific Research Publishing; 2020.

over narrow worldviews and self-interest. It awakens the aesthetic sense of human life, encouraging broader perspectives, objectivity, rationality, and relevant responses to pressing moral issues. In a world full of moral complexities, we struggle to cultivate a purposeful moral self. Our efforts to develop a more mature moral self in our personhood will always fall short of their potential. However, if we embrace the vision of aesthetics in all aspects of human life, self-evolution and moral awareness will naturally follow.

The aesthetic sense of human life that shapes our perception of the world is closely linked to the psycho-emotional and cognitive processes of higher-order personhood. Creating a better world relies on psycho-emotional conditions that positively influence behavior patterns. Modern psychology emphasizes that self-evolution improves psycho-emotional health and promotes behavioral change.[42] Moral consciousness, which results from self-evolution, acts as a pathway to a matured moral self and the psychosocial maturity of higher-order personhood.

We usually relate to people by identifying as liberals or conservatives, progressives or traditionalists, and, more commonly heard today, factualists or centrists – but not aestheticists. In our world, there seems to be a different baseline in moral values and attitudes, but in reality, people on both sides of the aisle are scared and trying to protect themselves from harm.

Evolutionary theorists argue that in the animal kingdom, the "harm-based mind" was a necessary survival trait. It was crucial for our early human ancestors during the initial phases of human evolution. Having a harm-based mind might have helped human development, but today, it hinders our ability for empathetic friendliness, cooperative mutuality, respectful tolerance, and peaceful coexistence.

---

[42] Kohrt B.A., et.al. Why we heal: The evolution of psychological healing and implications for global mental health. Clinical Psychology Review (Vol. 82); 2020

In modern society, people's harm-based thinking blocks opportunities for open dialogue and teamwork. This comes from ideological barriers created between individuals, fanatic groups, and nations. When we see ourselves as victims of those on the opposite side, we become closed off and unreceptive. Without self-improvement, we hold onto irrational thoughts and feelings. There is resistance to adopting a new view of the mature moral self, which is crucial for the psychosocial maturity needed to handle today's moral issues.

Without an appreciation for the aesthetic of human life, no one wants to believe they are simply victims of the mind's thought patterns shaped by the rationale and logic of the "fixed mindset" created by a static, rigid moral self. When we perceive that someone is trying to harm us, we shift into a defensive mode. As a result, people avoid dialogue and discussion, leading to disputes and hostility. Consequently, the loss is the transformative power of the mature moral self, which is essential for everyone to work toward a common goal in human life.

We can only create the right environment to develop the aesthetic sense of human life by facing our own fears and prejudices. This means we stop the automatic thought patterns of the other side, driven by our own destruction. It also involves cultivating the moral ability to be willing to engage in negotiations to find compromises. Essentially, this implies the "growth mindset" of individuals committed to self-evolution and redefining their moral framework. When traditional moral ideals are prioritized over the aesthetic sense of human life, the rigid, weak, or underdeveloped moral self dominates one's moral structure.

Only the mature moral self and psychosocial maturity serve as means to reach compromises. The aesthetic sense of human life can support the development of the moral self, making it predictable across all circumstances, personal conditions, and social environments, while remaining aligned with the individual's moral identity. It helps people prioritize a mature moral self within their work self-concept and self-identity. In modern times, meaningful coexistence requires us to develop a sense of self that promotes mutual understanding and cooperation. When the principle of human solidarity is central to one's work self-concept and self-identity, we engage in a meaningful human existence. Then, we strive to live with others in unity, mutuality, and reciprocity through a coherent vision of humanity.

We live in a complex, constantly changing, and challenging world, and collaborating is equally intricate, daunting, and confusing; however, it is a vital necessity if we are to bring the much-needed "light" to these times. We do not need the heat of tempers and hostilities that destroy what is truly human in us and weaken the spirit of unity and cooperation for meaningful coexistence. Instead, we need to nurture the aesthetic sense of human life and practice patience to understand the moral chaos in the world, which is linked to the thinking patterns of each person's moral self. Navigating these times requires wisdom, prudence, and sound judgment at the individual, collective, and institutional levels. We become victims of our fears and prejudices when driven by irrationality and emotional reactions.

The main pillars of meaningful coexistence are respect and dignity. The fundamental respect owed to a human isn't always recognized, though. These pillars form the moral foundation for the empathy and courtesy necessary to create relationship patterns that promote human solidarity. They set the moral tone for intentional collaboration and a shared vision of a unified humanity. Social integration and cohesion rely on these pillars. We often struggle to maintain this, and when these pillars are undermined, we alter the moral framework for meaningful coexistence in society. However, this is exactly what happens when we swing too far between polarized thinking in our efforts to address problems and challenges in modern human life.

The potential "gift" we can be to one another to unify humanity remains unwrapped when people are caught in the frenzy of polemics that destroy it. In today's world, with diverse perspectives, we have a responsibility to approach moral disagreements carefully and thoughtfully, as they impact global peace and the creation of a new world order. It depends on recognizing each other as gifts. This means everyone needs to consciously consider what divides and unites us. If we want to approach life with compassion, tolerance, and respect, we must foster an appreciation for human life, cultivate a mature moral self, and develop psychosocial maturity in all.

The commitment to work together toward the shared goal of a healthier humanity and a better world is deeply rooted in mutual trust and understanding. However, we cannot trust people if we do not know them. And, we cannot truly know people if we do not allow ourselves to see and experience them for who they really are. The way we learn about people in modern society is often through the generalizations made about them.

The typical way we see each other involves factors like gender, race, ethnicity, religious affiliation, sexual orientation, occupation, social status, public identity, talents, virtues, failures, and flaws. This is a lazy mental shortcut we use to judge people. It takes effort to resist the tendency to view others as just a collection of traits. The world we live in calls for a mindset that goes beyond stereotypes, which can only be achieved through a deeper understanding of human life.

Neuroscience demonstrates that we are hardwired for biases and prejudices.[43] As humans, biases and prejudices are common and greatly influence how we think and act. When the moral self lacks a sense of aesthetics, we fail to recognize the biases that shape our perceptions of others. We remain unaware of the prejudiced thinking patterns imprisoning our minds. As a result, we are less likely to be seen as trustworthy and as partners dedicated to building a healthier humanity and a new world order.

---

[43] Blink, GM. The Power of Thinking Without Thinking. Little, Brown and Company; 2005.

What makes us human is our ability to recognize true humanity in each other. We must work to overcome tendencies to fear, hate, or ostracize others. We need to develop the ability to see the full humanity of those around us. Inclusion, collaboration, and participation of everyone—regardless of ideological differences—are essential, unlike disbanding, exclusion, and non-participation driven by a divide-and-conquer mentality. These are central to the core principle of human solidarity. Mutual tolerance, respect, and honor are vital for experiencing human solidarity.

Evolutionary anthropologists tell us that, genetically, humans have evolved to live interdependently with one another. And that, genetically, can best adapt to human life by living in an environment of interdependency. We are wired to belong to one another. When this occurs, it characterizes the higher-order personhood manifested through the behaviors of the mature moral self and psychosocial maturity. If we are purposeful in collaborating to unify humanity, then there is a need to address the root causes of the deteriorating moral environment in the world. The rampant injustices, inequalities, and evildoings in our world hint at how self-seeking we are and how poorly we belong to one another.

In today's world, our experience of higher-order personhood is declining. Instead, people's personhood is often defined by egotism, self-centeredness, and utilitarian individualism. The aesthetic value of human life is fundamentally driven by higher-order personhood, which we lack. Cooperative mutuality, interdependence, and meaningful coexistence rely on people's higher-order personhood. To genuinely accept and value what is truly human in one another, without exceptions or expectations, higher-order personhood must be acknowledged.

In modern society, we often struggle to empathize and tend to react impulsively with outrage, frequently seeking revenge for wrongs. However, while we believe it is right to justify punishment when someone harms us, we also understand that we should not hurt others in return. We all have an internal sense of what is humane. We uniquely possess higher intellectual and emotional abilities that allow us to develop empathy and friendliness toward everyone, even our enemies. We experience the beauty of human life only when the mature moral self helps us see what it means to be human in others and stops the mindset driven by revenge.

Humans, unlike the rest of the animal kingdom, are not only endowed with a moral nature but can also develop their moral abilities. What sets us apart is our capacity to intentionally and volitionally refrain from harming others. Neuroscience demonstrates that the human brain is wired to protect both ourselves and others, even when the other is unrelated or hostile to us. There is neuroscientific evidence of uniquely human brain mechanisms that trigger protective behaviors.[44]

Primarily, the aesthetic sense of human life enhances our feeling of belonging to one another in all situations. It fosters a stronger connection to the "otherness" within us. The aesthetic sense can help people go beyond the boundaries that separate them. Without a moral sense and motivation centered on otherness, we create a life that is difficult, painful, and miserable for each other. As a result, this also makes our existence painfully lonely. We all need to develop a higher level of personhood to pursue greater ideals and purposes for our human life.

When the sense of self develops together with an appreciation for human life, language always has the power to heal and bring people together. The goal is simply to do what benefits the common good. Words are vital in creating a healthier humanity and a better world. In these difficult times, the moral self urges us to shape our language accordingly. We need to communicate with others in mind, embracing inclusive perspectives of mutual care and

---

[44] Coan, J. Familiarity promotes the blurring of self and other in the neural representation of threat. Journal of Social Cognitive and Affective Neuroscience, Vol 8; 2013

support to unite humanity. Too often, we mistake coherence for unification and use divisive language to create separation. This mistake is common among politicians, religious leaders, social celebrities, and other public figures who lack an aesthetic appreciation of human life. We falter when our everyday interactions are influenced by stereotypes, biases, and fears.

The ideas we introduce into the world shape the kind of society and humanity we develop. The human essence, viewed through the metaphysical, makes all people inherently truth-seekers. A unified view of humanity sees us as truth-seekers who also claim the truth. However, with an aesthetic appreciation of human life, careful and thoughtful truth assertions recognize that others, in good faith, may perceive the truth differently than we do. When sharing our perceptions, we should consider others' perspectives. To achieve shared understanding, we must not dismiss another person's truth. The aesthetic aspect of human life mainly guides the mature moral self, helping us recognize and honor the many nuances within truth.

Today, many public policies that restrict freedom of expression and speech in the name of national security stem from a distorted view of aesthetics in human life. They, in fact, deny people the right to express their moral self. Censoring others' moral self in the pursuit of truth effectively suppresses the truth itself. However, when objective truth is clear, we act knowingly with a mature moral self to uphold human dignity in all circumstances. This arises from a moral sense rooted in the aesthetics of human life. It is the aesthetics of human life, along with the straightforward objective truth, that motivates us to do everything possible to support fundamental principles of life, such as interdependence and human solidarity, which enable society to function optimally.

The most divisive moral and socio-political issues always stem from an inconsistent moral foundation within people—the fragile and inflexible moral self. Without moral awareness, the moral self is susceptible to the influences of personality and temperament. While truth can be hard to find, moral awareness in individuals is not.

We all need the aesthetic sense of human life to unlock the dormant potential of moral human nature. This potential arises from our innate moral capacities and human abilities necessary for psychosocial maturity in the postmodern world. The aesthetic sense of human life helps us stay focused and purposeful while respecting each person's inherent human dignity, worth, true self-identity, and full humanity. For genuine resolution of problems and challenges in our world, the aesthetic sense of human life is more effective than the norms and ideals of moral systems. It highlights that moral consciousness, a mature moral self, and high-level personhood are essential.

The aesthetic sense of human life relates to the potential of a person's moral self to develop the understanding and motivation needed for tolerance of differences, inclusiveness, respect, honor, and the pursuit of higher life ideals. Everyone has an innate moral capacity to go beyond self-interest and to sacrifice personal gain in order to prevent harm to others. This requires the higher-level personhood associated with a mature moral self and the psychosocial maturity necessary for us to be greater than ourselves. Higher-order personhood provides us with the credentials that demonstrate welcoming egalitarianism in how we treat others. The aesthetic sense of human life encourages behaviors that uphold respect for human dignity and coexistence without prejudice. Today, the visible positive benefits of this aesthetic sense, seen in some, serve as a reminder that society holds untapped potential that individuals must activate to live together as a unified and coherent humanity.

When reflecting on the deep human suffering caused by moral illness in today's world, the aesthetic sense of human life promotes the development of a mature moral self and psychosocial maturity in higher-order personhood, which are vital for addressing this challenge. Inspired by higher-order personhood, the aesthetic sense of human life helps fight against inhumanity in our world. It engages life through moral clarity, the purposefulness of the mature moral self, empathetic friendliness, psychosocial maturity, and especially, the vision of coherence that unites humanity.

Our pursuit of an aesthetic appreciation of human life occurs through positive imagination within our inner selves. This process mainly involves reflecting on the long trajectory of human history, which echoes the suffering and pain experienced in one's own life. It helps foster thoughts and behaviors that form the foundation of our aesthetic understanding of human existence.

CONCLUSION

The unique purpose and meaning of human life lie in the moral self of personhood. The moral self is always a tool used in the pursuit of happiness for everyone. Today, the strength and influence of the mature moral self surpass that of the state, religion, armies, and governments.

The moral self of personhood is a vital indicator and fundamental part of a society's well-being, resilience, and stability. The moral environment of a society reflects the moral self of its people. The moral self of individuals, rather than the moral ideals outlined in moral systems, religious traditions, or legal statutes, shapes the moral environment. Improving the moral environment of society relies on each person actively working to rebuild moral identity and restore the moral self.

It can be said that in modern society, people's moral framework lacks the necessary moral sensitivity and rationality to overcome destructive thinking and behavioral patterns. The socially binding moral self produces irrelevant and ineffective moral responses, some of which even have harmful consequences.

In a constantly changing world, especially in the moral realm, effective and relevant responses are shaped by understanding broader social, cultural, and historical contexts. They require that the moral self focus on the present. Concepts like altruism, other-oriented thinking, interdependence, human solidarity, and meaningful coexistence reflect a moral self of personhood that is different from one subjected to external coercion of normative morality.

A society functions well when individuals embody mature moral selves in their daily lives. The moral climate of society emphasizes how the moral self of personhood is often perceived as incompatible with otherness, interdependence, human solidarity, and coexistence—all of which are essential for improving humanity's well-being and caring for the planet.

In today's world, pursuing happiness requires us to dedicate ourselves to something beyond personal interests. Unfortunately, more people seem indifferent to the well-being of others. We don't see others' happiness as benefiting ourselves or the broader community. We fail to recognize that the main moral obligation in human life is to protect everyone's basic rights.

No one deserves to be treated as less than human, no matter how negatively they are viewed or judged. For most of us, our moral self isn't centered on the question of how to be human in the world. We often overlook the principles of interdependence and human solidarity as we try to improve the moral environment around us. We tend to forget to prioritize higher-level personhood as a way to grow in our humanity.

We do not regard the concept of moral disease when it comes to wrongdoings, heinous behaviors, corruption, or dangerously harmful evil acts. Despite advances in medical and health sciences, there isn't enough emphasis on moral disease as a health issue in healthcare and treatment. We do not view moral disease as a public health crisis.

The widespread issue of moral diseases, a significant health concern in our world, negatively affects humanity. Today, humanity must focus more on the moral well-being of individuals and society than on any other human activity. This emphasis will promote understanding of how moral responsibility and free will should work together for the common good, helping to positively shape the moral environment globally.

The moral climate in our world is not primarily due to failing moral standards or the guiding principles of people's moral selves, but rather due to a lack of development in moral awareness. There is a widespread agreement that the moral self plays a key role in encouraging prosocial behaviors, reducing antisocial actions, sharing responsibilities, and resisting the risk factors of catastrophic threats facing humanity. However, the complexity of moral issues in human life cannot be fully addressed by moral norms, ideals, and laws alone to ensure the relevance of the moral self in all moral situations.

The feeling of delusional self-identity is common in modern society. This is because we judge the success or failure of the moral self based on traditional morality standards, rather than higher-order personhood. Usually, the tool used to assess the moral self is moral conscience, not moral consciousness. As a result, people tend to be indifferent to the integrity, authenticity, and autonomy of personhood. This neglect worsens personality disorders, which are now more problematic and threatening to society than in previous generations.

Higher-order personhood is becoming increasingly rare in our world. In postmodern times, destructive cultural influences hinder the pursuit of higher ideals and life purposes. We follow strangers' virtual realities and imitate people we don't know well. We admire social celebrities, many of whom display moral decline, as role models and guides for developing a moral self and authentic personhood.

Without the higher-order personhood, the damaging cultural forces of the postmodern world are driving humanity toward total destruction. Without a mature moral self, we cannot prevent the unforeseen consequences of our collective moral choices, actions, and behaviors.

Humanity must repair the moral self. This requires each person to engage in self-improvement to achieve higher levels of personhood. The development of the moral self can happen through either moral conscience or moral consciousness. The moral self that guides everyday actions comes from either moral consciousness or moral conscience.

The mature moral self and psychosocial maturity of higher-order personhood can only result from moral consciousness, which develops in a person through self-evolution. Moral consciousness plays an active role in the regenerative design of moral identity and the rehabilitation of the moral self. The maturity of the moral self will come from engaging in self-evolution and adopting higher-order personhood.

No single person can create a healthier humanity and a better world alone. The effort to close the significant gaps in our modern society highlights the collective nature of this work. When each of our lives aligns with a shared mission—pursuing the common good, fostering human solidarity, and building a healthier humanity and better world—we take the right steps to overcome divisions, hatred, and harmful mindsets.

The vision for the 21st-century world should be one where everyone takes responsibility for creating conditions that allow all people to pursue happiness. Whether we realize it or not, everyone wants to fit into the world in a meaningful way. It's not enough just to hold ideals of a free world and freedom for all; people also need the psycho-emotional resources that enable them to experience this reality. This requires us to develop a deeper aesthetic understanding of human life.

Creating a better world means not turning away from suffering and doing everything we can to ease it when it occurs. We cannot ignore the devastation faced by people whose lives have been upended by tragedies not of their own making but caused by others. Confronting the deep cries of human suffering in our world and reflecting on our own moral integrity often helps us develop a radical vision of building a world for others, which we also long for ourselves.

The world does not improve merely by promoting ideas of moral change; instead, it advances through models we can imitate to foster moral growth. We will not overcome difficult times for humanity if we are afraid to stand alone or be different with our mature moral selves. Although global culture often seems dedicated to the gradual erosion of people's moral character, we must all intentionally work to contribute positively and create beneficial changes in each other's lives. This will only happen when people's personhood is enriched with an aesthetic sense of human life, expressed through the mature moral self and the psychosocial development of higher-order personhood.